GONE MAD
a true story

DEMENTIA, FAMILY TREACHERY, AND LEGAL INSANITY

BY CAROL PENDERGRASS

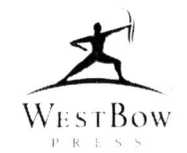

WestBow
PRESS

Copyright © 2010 Carol Pendergrass

All rights reserved. No part of this book may be used or reproduced by any means, graphic, electronic, or mechanical, including photocopying, recording, taping or by any information storage retrieval system without the written permission of the publisher except in the case of brief quotations embodied in critical articles and reviews.

This book is a work of non-fiction. Unless otherwise noted, the author and the publisher make no explicit guarantees as to the accuracy of the information contained in this book and in some cases, names of people and places have been altered to protect their privacy.

WestBow Press books may be ordered through booksellers or by contacting:

WestBow Press
A Division of Thomas Nelson
1663 Liberty Drive
Bloomington, IN 47403
www.westbowpress.com
1-(866) 928-1240

Because of the dynamic nature of the Internet, any Web addresses or links contained in this book may have changed since publication and may no longer be valid. The views expressed in this work are solely those of the author and do not necessarily reflect the views of the publisher, and the publisher hereby disclaims any responsibility for them.

ISBN: 978-1-4497-0214-4 (sc)
ISBN: 978-1-4497-0216-8 (hc)
ISBN: 978-1-4497-0215-1 (e)

Library of Congress Control Number: 2010927358

Printed in the United States of America

WestBow Press rev. date: 7/19/2010

This book is dedicated to my beloved husband Don,
To caregivers everywhere,
And to the Lewy Body Dementia Association

www.lbda.org

Contents

Acknowledgements ix

Introduction xi

Part I 1

Looking Back	3
Second Chances	10
Frank	22
The Quarry, 1998	26
Meanwhile …	29
The Descent Begins	31
Matters of the Heart	34
2006	41
The Other Carols	52
Carol Who Works at the Office	56
Home	61
Laughter and Despair 2007	66
The Diagnosis	69
The Sound of a Dropping Shoe	72
The Law	84
A Moment of Clarity	93
The Cuckoo's Nest	97
How Much Worse Can It Get?	104
Show Me the Money	107
The Sun Goes Down	109

Part II 119

"Surprise!" — 121
Alone — 126
Accusations — 130
The Electric Chair — 132
Stand in Line — 136
Reunited with My Husband — 141
Is There No Peace Anywhere? — 145
Finding a New Normal — 154
God Speaks to Me — 158
No Laws, No Justice — 161
Waiting on the Train — 165
"It Is What It Is" — 170

Part III 177

Discovery — 179
Enough — 187
Visitation — 189
Crossing the Borders — 192
What Was Meant for Evil — 195
March 2008 — 199
Lessons — 202
Death Do Us Part — 219
My Personal Living Will — 229

10 Things You Should Know about LBD 231

Acknowledgements

Writing this book was therapy in the midst of a situation in which I had completely lost control of my life. I am so thankful for my family and friends who stepped into the situation with me to love and protect me; to pray for me and encourage me.

I thank Don for telling me to "write it down."

Foremost, I thank my son Rob, and my granddaughter Erin for loving me and giving peace and security to my life; my brothers and sisters who cried with me and held me together; and my Aunt Mary who was the most avid supporter of this book and believed in it from the beginning. Thanks to our many friends who supported me, read the book at different stages of writing, and offered valuable suggestions. I am most grateful for the work of my brother Mark D. Pendergrass who helped me in the writing of the book; who designed and developed the book cover, and put me in contact with the right people. And to my sister Rhandi who tirelessly worked as assistant, promoter and agent for the book. Without any one of these people in my life, this book would not have happened. Special thanks to Gary, Joyce, Karen, Ken, Gary and Colene, Sharon and Kelly, and Warren and JoAnn. My longtime friend, Charles L. Stanley *CFP ChFC AIF* reviewed the parts of the book on Trusts and life planning and gave excellent information and counsel.

A special acknowledgment to Joyce White who took care of Don in the nursing home, when I could not. I am most grateful for her kindness to me as well as her loving care of Don.

I want to acknowledge the love of God in my life, and the thankfulness I have for His presence and goodness to me. I am thankful to my parents for the godly home which was the incubator of my faith. I am thankful for the joy with which I have been blessed.

I am thankful for the many minutes, hours, days, and years that I got to spend with Don. He was the love of my life. Our love transcended all else that came our way. For your love, and for every minute I got to be with you, "Thank you, Don."

For caregivers everywhere I offer prayer every day. I acknowledge the sacrifices you make. LBD is an insidious disease which is unbelievably cruel both to its victims and to the caregivers. Until recently I did not realize that Don's actions were classic LBD symptoms, and that what I have described in the book is the pattern for sufferers of LBD. Caregivers are heroes who devote themselves in the face of the abuse this disease brings. With this book my hope is that caregivers will feel appreciated and validated, and that through it they will find help and encouragement. After Don's death I discovered the Lewy Body Dementia Association. I am grateful for the work they are doing in bringing awareness of this common but little known, complex disease, and for giving a format for discussion and interaction between caregivers through Facebook.

Don's and my hope for our life together was that we could make a difference in just one person's life. My wish for this book is that it will fulfill that hope and in some way make the life of every reader just a little better.

Introduction

Somewhere high in my family tree sits Louisa May Alcott. Although I would love to claim from the gene pool her way with words, that ship sailed without me long ago. Aunt Louisa wrote novels; I write Post-it notes. At least that was about the extent of it for me until something happened in my life that would not fit on a three-by-three-inch slip of paper. Something I needed to write down for myself; something I hoped to understand in the writing; something that I've discovered upon writing could be of help to those who might one day find themselves in a similar predicament. Of *Little Women*, Louisa said, "The characters were drawn from life, which gives them whatever merit they possess, for I find it impossible to invent anything half so true or touching as the simplest facts with which everyday life supplies me," and I follow her in that—writing about what I know best: my family, and what actually happened to us.

This book will not be the great American novel, eloquently written. If only it were fiction; then I could say good-bye to the characters, close the cover, and leave them in their tome. Because my story is not fiction but astoundingly true, and now I know it could happen to anyone, it is a story that must be told.

Fundamental Christians are not known to believe in Purgatory. Once, I didn't either. Purgatory: that hauntingly dark realm between this world and the next, where souls are waylaid on their way to the peace of eternity. To be refined? To pay for their sins? To wander aimlessly until they have paid an undefined price to pass through the final gate? Whatever its purpose, my husband and I went there together. He did not come back.

We were totally unprepared for this experience because it happened in this life, while we were both still breathing. We found ourselves groping for something familiar or secure. We were constantly faced with obstacles we could never have imagined before. This was a place filled with beings that were foreign and terrible; a place where the living and the dead seemed to cross paths simultaneously. So strange was it that, as Dante described it, even the sun was not in its rightful place, casting shadows that were terrible, and grew more so every day.

Most of the time I was able to walk in and out of the door to that world at will, but for my husband, it became his final residence on earth. There was only one way for him to escape, and he had not yet come to that gateway. When I would emerge into the light, the world was as it had always been. The sun warmed me. The sheer sanity of life, like an easy chair, would embrace me in her soft arms, and I would feel peace—until those two worlds would again merge into one as I was drawn by my love for my husband back into the dark place of his mind. To be with him, I walked through that door again and again, completely unprepared for the barrage of demons we would ultimately face on both sides. Here, there were no walls to keep out the rabid animals or the visiting dead. There were no doors to keep at bay the intruders who stole from us both body and spirit. There were no rules or laws, which must exist if any world is to be kept in balance.

I have a story to tell that every married couple in America should hear. It will take many slips of paper to tell it through to the end. But I have found the courage to write it down. And I pray that it will serve as an instruction manual for those who one day find themselves in that Purgatory from which I have emerged. Had I known what I know now, many nightmarish pitfalls could have been avoided; many demons vanquished. There are those who will say that this could not possibly happen in a country of laws and provisions; where the sanctity of marriage is held in high esteem. Those who lived this story with us say, "But that can't happen," or "They can't do that." But of course it can happen, and it did happen, and it will happen again.

PART ONE

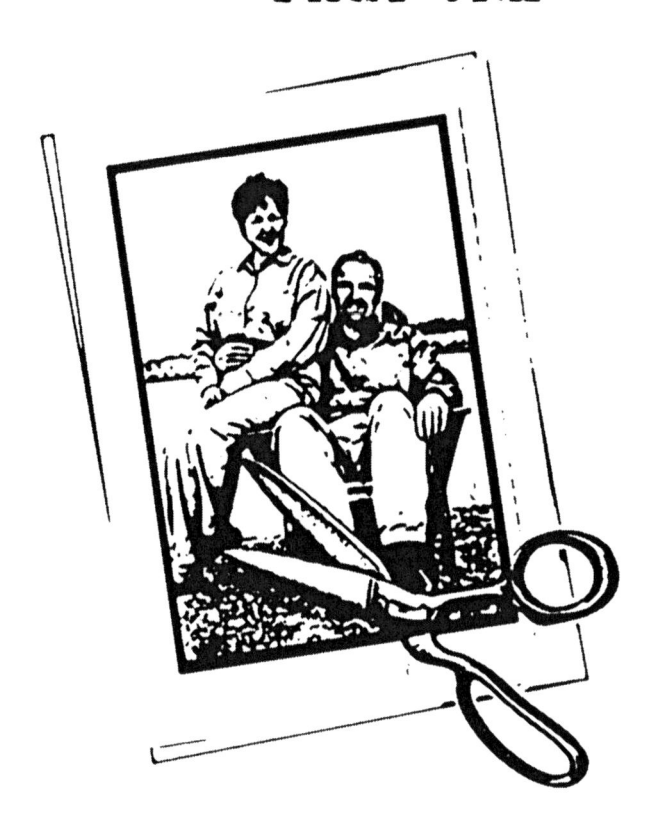

Looking Back

I'm just an average woman with the majority of my life behind me. I've had my share of success in the business world, but like a lot of postwar baby boomers, I consider my greatest accomplishment to be the family that I have made: a son and two grandchildren, an eighteen-year marriage to a wonderful man, and a warm relationship with his five children from a former marriage and his nine grandchildren. Family is the basis for all else in my life. It is noble, stabilizing, an anchor for the body and soul. It is that best part of God we share with one another while on this earth. I could never have imagined that at a time when I should be celebrating the fruit of my labor, when grandchildren should be crawling up on my lap for just one more story, or our children should be calling to seek out wisdom in the wake of hard-won mutual respect, that suddenly all that I hold dear, all that I have worked for in life, could be utterly destroyed: my family, my marriage, my reputation, my future. Though I have always felt somewhat in control of my life, something was put into motion that I could not stop. Something that I did not foresee; something that, frankly, no one deserves to have happen to them; something that I hope to help others avoid. But I'm getting ahead of myself. For before that "something" happened to me, my life was wonderful beyond all my romantic dreams.

My husband, Don, was an exceptional man. The first time I saw him, he seemed to completely fill the hallway where he stood.

It was as though no one else could fit into the room. It took a moment to realize it was his presence, not his stature, which filled all the space around him. At almost six feet tall, his shoulders were extraordinarily straight and broad. I wanted to put my hands on his shoulders to see if they were real. I thought him not particularly handsome, but he had a very interesting, rugged face and teasing eyes. Later in our relationship, I would amuse him by saying that he looked like a tomcat that had been around the block a few times. He had great character in his face, an intensity that could be disarming. He was arrogant and cocky, and grossly self-assured. I thought, *This is the straightest man I have ever seen.* He exuded power and control. He was all business; I thought, *Here is a man who fits the idiom "all work and no play."*

From our first meeting, he courted me relentlessly. As cynical as I had become through a devastating divorce, I was no longer the starry-eyed girl I had once been. Winning me over would take some time, but for Don, it was a foregone conclusion. As he often said, for him it was "love at first sight." He got me in his sights, and it wasn't long before I was caught in his magnetism. To me, he was vintage Clint Eastwood: cool, sexy, fearless, and always in control.

We had each experienced marriage, children, disappointment, divorce, and a sense of the old Peggy Lee song, *Is That All There Is?* to life.

I can't say that Don robbed the cradle when he married me, but there was a definite age difference between us. In 1947, the year I was born, Don was climbing up onto a tractor to help plow the fields on his father's farm. In 1965, the year I graduated from high school, Don had already graduated college, married, had four children, and was senior vice president of a bank. In July of 1969, when my only son was born, Don had his fifth and last child. That same week, somewhere above our heads, a man walked on the moon, the same moon that shone on both of us but in our separate worlds.

Don was raised in the panhandle of Oklahoma. I call his family the Oklahoma Ewings. They even have a J.R. and a Bobby. Don was the youngest of three boys. The family ranch was large and successful, but Don had different ambitions. He left the farm, went to college, and started a career in the big city. But you know what they say about the farm and the boy. He made me think of my father, who had died years before: a strong man who knew that life came from sacrifice and the hard work of a man's own hands. My grandparents farmed in the Oklahoma panhandle where I spent many summers of my life, and Don and I seemed to be connected by the roots that ran under the red dirt. My father always said the red of Oklahoma's dirt came from the blood poured into it. Don was older than me by ten years; I loved his maturity, his rugged good looks, his callused hands—hands that knew what it meant to work hard and get the job done; hands into which I could entrust my life. I knew that with him I would always be secure, loved, and protected. Don was a force of nature. He could will things to happen, and they happened. He was self-confident, self-disciplined. If he set his mind to something, it would take divine intervention to deter him. He had a Mensa-level IQ and always seemed to be several steps ahead of everyone around him. His philosophies were simple, his beliefs deep, and he found value in every person he met. I loved him for all of those things and for the complexities of this man I could never fully know.

With me, Don was never overbearing. We both had strong personalities, and at times, our opinions collided. But Don's gentle way of conversation and reasoning left no room for anger or frustration. More often than not, I was the one proven wrong, but I would press the issue anyway, rhetorically betting everything I owned on whether what we saw across the lake was a dead duck or a stone! Whether on politics, religion, ethics, you name it … we would challenge one another like iron sharpens iron. And in the end, whether it was a rock or a dead duck, we were always bonded together by one intangible gift: a relationship that allowed for differing thoughts and opinions, no matter how silly they might be. He even "got" my dark sense of humor. With Don, I felt completely safe to be exactly who I was.

If you put a match to dry wood, you get ashes. That's the chemistry of an imperfect world. But Don and I were like the burning bush that Moses saw in the desert; like a spirit-born flame, our passion burned hot but never burned out. We were blessed with the kind of mutual zeal for life, love, and family that seemed to give a perfect balance to life.

Don had an air about him that was comforting to some, unnerving to others; a formidable man; one to be reckoned with, especially in the business world. He had the ambition and ability to carry out any goal he set for himself. He had an amazing ability to take a bad situation and suddenly flip it so that he was totally in charge. He loved a challenge. He was a risk-taker. But risk always means that there is plenty of room for failure—the very fact that makes it so exciting.

By the time we met, Don had left the senior vice presidency of the bank and was involved with real estate investment. He was happy to be out of the bureaucracy and away from the world of striped suits and silk ties. He'd had enough of traveling, lecturing, auditing, granting or turning down loans, and resolving conflicts. No more days that started at 4:00 am and ended at 10:00 pm for him. Don took well to the casual life. Although he owned his business, he would often say, "I'm just the maintenance man." He never needed anyone else's confirmation to know who he was. More often than not, you'd see him in cowboy boots, a well-worn pair of jeans, a T-shirt, and a denim jacket, carrying a battered briefcase that would never quite close. But running your own life brings the possibility for considerably greater risks. And there would be trouble on the horizon that threatened to destroy him.

Don loved to put deals together, not so much for the money as for the thrill of the danger involved. Don and his nephew, Frank, had grown up together on the cattle ranch in Oklahoma, and the two of them had always been close. Frank is what you'd call an authentic cowboy. As I heard the story, in the 1980s, he and Don entered into a "no-lose" cattle venture, with Frank managing the cattle in Jackson Hole, Wyoming. When it came time for them to go to market, Frank called Don and informed his uncle that the cattle were missing. In that one simple phone call, Don assumed the total loss of over a quarter of a million dollars. Frank, having literally lost a fortune in cattle as well as a fourth wife in divorce, moved to the same Kansas town where Don had been living for several years. And though it seemed he had thoroughly botched up Don's life as well as his own, Frank was received with open arms.

With the failed cattle deal and the debt hanging over him, Don began sinking into a deep depression. Together, Don and Frank began to indulge in a lifestyle of bars and carousing. Don was swiftly losing himself. His marriage ended during that time, and his disappointment over failure was more than he could cope with. He could hear his father's words echo constantly in his head: "Death is preferable to bankruptcy." He began to contemplate suicide. Often, Don would recount the story of how divine intervention had spared him at the last minute. One day, with his gun on the floorboard of his pickup, he set out for the family farm to end his life. Like George Bailey in *It's a Wonderful Life*, he had reached the conclusion that he was worth more dead than alive. And like George, God got involved, as Don's truck was broadsided by another vehicle on a country road. No one was badly injured, but the collision jarred more than nuts and bolts. Don was miraculously awakened from his depression and began to emerge into the light of life once again. After that, Don never hid the fact of his depression and eagerly listened to other men who were going through similar circumstances, ever encouraging them to hold onto hope.

As for me, I was the proverbial "Church Lady." All of my life I had found my identity in the church, and even as an adult, I still attended and volunteered my time at the church our family had been a part of all my life. Though I had moved away from Kansas a few times, I always found my way back to that same little congregation upon each return. Things were constant there; the pews were clearly defined by the families that had been filling them for decades.

In the late 1970s, my life took an unexpected turn when my marriage of thirteen years dissolved. A life of stability and predictability suddenly began to spiral out of control. My husband filed for divorce. In those days, there was such a stigma in our church surrounding divorce that I doubted I could survive it and remain in the church with my dignity intact. I had a ten-year-old son, who was my passion. He and I left our home as my ex-husband moved in his new family. The volunteer work I did at the church was terminated, and I had to search for a paying job. My decision to keep our family affairs private, along with my ex-husband's accusations, made me fair game for all the gossip a close-knit church could muster. Stripped of all leadership, I watched in despair, as my identity and integrity were lost. I had no friends outside of the church, and at that time, my entire family was scattered across the map, leaving me virtually on my own for the first time in my life. With the exception of my son, I was completely alone.

My family wasn't nearby, and truly I'm not sure that I would have wanted them there. Everything and everyone I encountered seemed only to complicate a situation that I felt incapable of dealing with at the time. I was like a mother bear facing winter storms; I just wanted to take my cub and disappear into a cave and sleep away the harsh days ahead. But it was a long time till spring, so I found a job, moved into an apartment, and quietly proceeded to raise my son on my own.

Divorce for any reason brings a sickness of the soul that is long lasting. I wrestled with guilt and shame, and often I despaired, thinking I would not survive this sickness. I no longer knew who I was. Redefining oneself at any time of life is a daunting task, but I had no choice. I had to discover who I was outside of marriage and the church, and who I was going to be for the rest of my life. I laid out specific plans for my son and myself, making vows that would affect every aspect of our lives. I tried to obey God at every turn and listen to His wisdom. Eventually I began to gain some footing, taking pride in my accomplishments and learning to like myself once again. My father used to say, "If anyone has done it before, you can learn to do it, too." I held onto those words like scripture. If my dryer broke down, I turned it around, studied the manual, and fixed it myself. I repaired the toilet and changed the oil in my car. I was becoming empowered. In the business world, I began to make my way into better positions, earning more money and using it wisely. I was beginning to find my new self and move comfortably into my new life.

In our lives, there are defining moments when we make decisions that change the course of our future. Sometimes they just happen, and sometimes they are gifts offered by God. In 1979, I started working in an entry-level accounting position, making a whopping $3.25 an hour. By 1982, I was payroll manager for a large oil-drilling company, making good money and enjoying the perks of a wealthy business. But by Memorial Day of that year, when my son, Rob, was turning the worrisome age of thirteen and my mother was about to lose a second husband to cancer, God offered me a deal. My son needed me with him that summer, and my mother needed my help as her husband lay dying. I made a covenant with God that I would choose my family over my career; I had faith that when school started in the fall, and my mother's husband was buried, God would provide the gift of another job for me. As I locked up my house, and my son and I left for my mother's home in Oklahoma for the summer, I put my future in God's hands … right where He wanted me.

I was tempted with interesting job offers during those summer months but each wanted me to start working right away. When the position God wanted me to have came along, I was asked when I *wanted* to start, and so, in keeping with our covenant, I chose to start my new job on the same day school started in the fall. I knew it was a God-given job, but I did not know how far-reaching God's gifts could be! On the surface, it was nothing more than a position in a small office working for R. F. Roberts, an independent oil and gas producer. But I learned the oil business, from drilling to accounting, from a man who would bless me throughout the remainder of my life. He was my surrogate father; my mentor. Rob and I became an extension of his family, and after his death in 1996, I became administer of his trusts. I worked on his behalf for twenty-six years, and much of what I have, he blessed me with. That decision to do the right thing for my family and then wait on the fulfillment of God's end of the bargain changed the course of my future.

After my son graduated in 1987 and was on his own, I wanted to buy a house. My real estate broker was Don. Our love story began the moment we met.

Second Chances

Don and I were married on August 18, 1990. By this time, Don was deeply in debt, and he was determined to repay the bank every cent of the cattle loss. Of course, I was aware of his situation and also accepted it. We knew that together, we could overcome this and build a new life. I am not a thrill-seeker. In fact, I am known to be a "worst-case scenario" person—I think, *What would be the worst thing that could happen under the circumstances?* and make my decision based on whether I could live with that. We both knew our differing views on risk-taking could be a problem, so we determined to keep our investments separate. When we married, I said, "I won't ask how much you *make* if you don't tell me how much you *owe*!" That became our way of living financially, and it suited us. I made sure all of our living expenses were met, and Don paid down his debt and financed the real estate brokerage. We each kept our own accounts and trusted each other to take care of our respective obligations. We kept our finances separate and had absolutely no arguments over money or securities in our entire marriage.

Don and I carefully planned our lives together. We both had children and established family relationships that we hoped to integrate into one family. I respected the fact that Don's children had a mother, and it wasn't me. I thought the best I could hope for was to be accepted as the woman their father now loved and who made him happy because of my love for him. Before our marriage, we began to establish a relationship with each of his children and their mates. I felt totally accepted. I knew little about Don's first marriage. That relationship seemed to be off-limits for conversation, which was okay with me. Don respected her as the mother of his children, and that began and ended any conversation about them. Obviously, it was not a fulfilling marriage, and Don was away from home most of the time as the children grew up. Now he longed for fun and a social life with friends, which he never had time for in his previous marriage.

Don was uncharacteristically romantic with me. He wrote poetry and stories for me that were both hilariously funny and warmly touching. His gifts were rarely extravagant, but I often found a pair of earrings or a trinket on my car seat at the end of the workday, letting me know he was thinking about me throughout the day. Don shunned romantic holidays such as Valentine's Day because he didn't want romance to be dictated. One February, a week before Valentine's Day, a bouquet of flowers was delivered to me. And one bouquet was delivered every day for six more days. But on February 14, Valentine's Day, there were no flowers, nor any mention of it being anything special. He wanted to be sure I knew he loved me because *he* chose to love me, not because he was *supposed* to. Seldom did we ever celebrate any holiday with gifts, but we celebrated every other day of the year out of pure love. Even a trip to the grocery store was celebrated with whatever he could find that he thought would please me—a houseplant, a dish, or a book.

Don didn't like secrets, and I didn't like surprises. Early in our relationship, we decided no matter what the situation, we were on the same team, and there would be no secrets and no surprises. So we always told each other about surprise parties or little jokes that others were going to play. We were like counter-spies! We were always in on it together. We didn't even surprise each other at Christmas; Don would always tell me what he was getting me, and I got to enjoy the gift long before I opened it.

It was he who wanted to be married in a "little white church in the country." All the summer of 1990, we drove around the small, quaint towns of Kansas until Don spotted the church he wanted just outside of Hesston, Kansas. We were jealous of this long-awaited day. We told our families of our plans, but we went alone on a very hot day in August to the little white church, where we were married in a simple but joyful ceremony with only the minister and his wife, a neighboring farmer in from the fields for his lunch, and his dog as our witnesses. A few weeks later, we had a lovely reception at our home, and our families and all of our friends joined in celebrating our marriage. Don and I felt at the center of our own universe with the joining of our families.

Our first grandchild was born the year we were married. There would be ten more grandchildren to follow. I often felt part of a huge tree with leaves falling all around us. We were all a part of each other and as a family, we insulated each other from the world around us. We had six children, six mates, and soon eleven grandchildren.

I grew up in a very religious, slightly upper-middle-class, Ozzie-and-Harriet-style family with four kids. My dad wore suits to work each day, and my mother wore a dress with an apron to do the housework. We went to church Wednesday nights and twice on Sunday, and most of the days in between. We entertained ourselves and each other, and we knew how to have a party! We were a fun family. Nothing made us feel more successful than to make each other laugh, and we did that a lot. My siblings had all migrated back to Kansas with their families by the time Don and I married. When my family first met Don, they embraced him completely and came to love him as their brother. We all really *liked* each other, and we got together as often as we could for dinner, cards, games, or just conversation.

For me, where two or more were gathered together, there was a party! We had an open-door policy and a party for every occasion. On holidays, we would have what we called "orphan parties"; if you had no other plans, you could come on over and party with us. Of course, with our combined families, we had a large number, but Don and I made friends easily, and everyone we knew was invited into our family. Early in our marriage, it never bothered us to fill every inch of our little house with family and friends. Everyone seemed to look forward to our parties, and no one enjoyed them more than

Don and I. Don was learning to have fun—I think for the first time! He was game for about anything; his portrayal of Willie Nelson was his most famous. And the funniest was Don and Frank costumed as the Blues Brothers, cartwheeling and tumbling into the room. The partygoers went wild! When they began their rendition of *Rawhide* in their black suits and hats, a spontaneous throwing of food broke out, mimicking the movie. It was an unexpected show of enjoyment from Don's children that thrilled him, and me as well.

For Don's children, this was a new side of their dad. At first, I don't think they knew how to take this new father. I had little insight into how they were raised, or what interaction they had with their father growing up. Early on, I saw that Don had different standards for his own children than for others, and it was my opinion that he intentionally kept them at a distance. Any discussion of this ended quickly; I wasn't going to change anything, and his relationship with his children was not a hill I wanted to die on. However, I was aware that we had a completely different perspective on being married-with-children.

My son Rob and Don were close. Rob loved Don and respected him, and accepted him without reservation. They introduced themselves as father and son, and it always amused us when the response was, "I can tell. You look so much alike." They never corrected anyone.

Don and I often said, "With six kids, and six mates, if we planned well, we'd never have to hire anyone for anything again!" We had raised lawyers and nurses and builders and repairmen and even a car salesman, so we'd never even have to haggle for a car! And we said with this many kids, we would have no need for nursing home insurance ... we'd just spend one day a week with each one!

I remember many years ago in our church, some children began to attend from a large Asian family. I asked one of the children if he had an older sister named Lens, with whom I had attended high school. The child thought a minute and said, "I think we have *one of those*"! Sometimes I felt like that, with so many in our family. I always felt like a little person around Don's family. The boys were six feet, three inches to six feet, five inches, and the girls towered over my five-foot, two-inch frame by half a foot or more. Don's five children are, in birth order with their mates, Kate, a school psychologist, and her husband, Larry, a local car dealership service manager; Carla, a medical researcher, and her husband, James, a malpractice attorney; Doug, a corporate attorney, and his wife, Nancy, a nurse; Dale, a technician and single father of two; and Dennis and his wife, Shelly, who are both computer specialists. My son Rob is raising two children alone and owns a trim carpentry company. We had the bases covered!

Don and I, having raised our children to adulthood, were now focused on our own marriage; our second chance at life. We were still young; we had a measure of success and a lot of ambition. We hoped that we could be one big, happy family, but that was not our mission. We would leave relationships with our families up to them to define, and we would secure our marriage above all else. Don's children seemed to embrace me and said on occasion how good it was to see their father happy. As the grandchildren came along, they never saw Grandpa without me by his side. It was important to Don that the grandchildren know that "Grandma and Grandpa love each other." But Don's grandchildren seemed to have been told, "She's not your real grandmother," and they were never close or snuggly to me. As they grew older, I sometimes felt they saw me as just the woman Gramps shacked up with. I let them define my role with them. The reality is that Don's children have a mother; she has a love and a history with them that is spiritual and follows with the grandchildren. I had no desire to usurp her or try to take anything away from her, so my feelings were not hurt if I was not "Grandma." And I was not.

I wasn't good at reading Don's children. All highly intelligent, they were gamesmen, and I was never in on their mind games. The sons-in-law, James and Larry, were especially a mystery to me. Although there were moments of warmth between us through the years, I was mostly just a stranger in their midst. Don's kids were accepting of my son Rob, but it was obvious that they never included him. Like me, he was not one of them. Our grandchildren got along well. They called themselves "cousins." At that age, no one cares how they are related. My granddaughter, Erin, and Don's granddaughter, Amanda, were good friends and frequently stayed the night together with us or at each other's homes. All considered, we felt we had a well-blended family and were proud of the relationships that were formed.

In our first years of marriage, Don and I looked for some interest we could share in our spare time. I loved antiques and things that had a history. One day, I saw a picture in the paper of an antique birdcage that was being offered at an auction. Because we had a couple of lively canaries, I thought that birdcage was just what we needed for our home. Don was an old cattle rancher, and his father had taken him to cattle auctions from early childhood. At age ten, he was allowed to bid on and buy cattle for the family. Auctions were old hat to him; I had never been to one. So he took me to the auction to buy me the birdcage.

The auction was held in an old building that was smoky and smelly and crude. There were rows of wooden bleachers, which seemed to be the only place to sit. There were men with dirty clothes and cowboy boots, and big cigars. The odor of smoke from the cigars mixed with the smoke from the grill where hot dogs were being turned to a blackened-brown. Children were running unsupervised. I felt like we were at a county fair; the atmosphere was exciting. And they were selling some very odd things in a manner I couldn't keep up with.

And then the birdcage was brought up by a grimy old man, and every fiber in my body tensed like Mr. Toad when he caught his first sight of a car! I had to have it, but I had no idea how to get it. Before I could even clear my mind enough to tell Don that's what we came for, I heard the man shout, "Sold!" I looked at Don, confused and panicked—as they brought the birdcage into the bleachers and handed it to me. I literally stood up and asked aloud, "Did we get this?" The auctioneer stopped, smiled, and said in a long drawl, "Yes ma'am, you did," and then went on to the next item. I watched Don closely then, as only his index finger went up when he bought me an antique ring. And I was absolutely, without shame, hooked on auctions!

We went with an old friend of Don's to an auction in a town several hours away. I was anxious to get there because many lovely, Victorian-era things were being offered. We were late arriving, and the seats were all full. I found one lone seat near the back and took it, as I was afraid the men were not taking this seriously at all. My husband and his friend stood at the back against the wall. A beautiful dresser set of comb, brush, and mirror, still in its exquisite antique box, was brought to the block. It was my first time to bid alone. I wasn't sure how to do this, but I knew that set was going home with me! So I stood up and held my numbered paddle in the air as the bidding began. And I stood there. My paddle never went down and neither did I. Don and his friend were laughing at the back, as was everyone else at the auction, and they let me stand there until they heard "Sold!" and the set was brought to me.

And so it was that we found our "something to do together." We got on every antique auction list in a four-state area, and carefully planned our weekends to hit the ones of most interest, sometimes going between two or three auctions in the same day. We were like a well-oiled machine, working the auctioneers and crowds, and gained a reputation among the antique buyers of being a force to be reckoned with. Our colorful auction experiences became our greatest stories, and the most fun we could have ever imagined together. We always remembered the wonderful, odd characters we met, and every piece in our home has a wonderful story behind it. We were a pair of birds building our nest out of another generation's discards. We each had our passions: mine for laces and rich fabrics with hundred-year-old fringe, and Don, for me. Many times, I would bid up to what I had decided I could pay for something and quit bidding, only to hear my number called out as Don continued to bid for me. Several times, my surprise stopped the auction as the bidders clapped over my good fortune. The auctioneers loved to see us coming and catered to us. We occasionally took my mother with us to out-of-town auctions. Once, she and I decided to bid on an exquisite antique tea set. When the bidding went past my limit, we were disappointed. When my number was called out as the winning bid and my mother realized that Don had bought it for me, at that moment she fell head-over-heels in love with my husband, and believe me, he could do no wrong from then on.

I was drawn like a magnet to odd things nobody else wanted. They never sold for much, so I would bid on the lone piece of china from a broken set; sepia pictures with no one left to look at them; a hand mirror separated from the comb and brush; an antique salt shaker that had lost its mate long ago. I called them my "widows."

We traveled to farm auctions, estate auctions, auctions on mountaintops, and auctions in barns. We stood in mud, snow, rain, and cow poop; sweltered; and froze. We loved the beautiful and unusual things we bought, especially the surprises we many times found in the bottom of boxes or hidden in books, and we loved the joy of doing it together. After a while, we accumulated so much stuff that we needed to either quit going or find an outlet. After doing a lot of homework on the resale business and a lot of planning, we opened a small shop in a quaint area of our city. There was no shop of its kind at that time. For years, country décor had been the fad, but I saw a change to Victorian on the horizon. Our merchandise was unusual and rare: small decorative Victorian items and accessories; lamps and rugs; laces and linens; antique jewelry; hats, gloves, hankies, and vintage clothing. I took on a partner, who taught needle arts in the shop such as tatting, crocheting, and silk ribbon embroidery. We had classes for children and adults, and the classes were always full. As a result of the shop, my partner became a published needle arts creator and a sought-after seminar instructor.

The shop was unusual, and we knew the articles we sought to sell were for a particular type of person. The name for our little shop needed to be almost a dare to indulge in what we had to sell. (I thought about "This Ain't K-Mart" but figured I'd get sued.) There was a card that surfaced at that time for women who dared to be different about "wearing purple" as an expression of oneself. Don and I played with the words and decided to call the shop "Wear Purple Victorian Shop." And it worked. We were a decade ahead of time, as there is now a very large nationwide "Red Hat Society" based upon the "Wear Purple" concept.

Don and I continued with our own businesses, ran the store, and every weekend traveled to auctions buying for the shop. We felt we were about as fulfilled and happy as we could be. When you work together all day and then go home together at night, you really have to be friends, and we were the best of friends. We had the shop for three years and then found that the quality of Victorian merchandise we wanted was falling. In those three years, antique malls (flea market venues) became popular. The vendors had no overhead. Competition was getting ruthless, and we decided unless we compromised our inventory, we should just quit. We both felt it was time to get back to growing our real estate business.

As ambitious people do, Don branched out when the opportunity presented itself and began to manage rental properties. He started a property management company that grew to about sixty residential homes and a few commercial properties. He liked the interaction with his clients and was happiest when faced with a challenging situation. He remembered the years of sitting in front of the radio listening to President Roosevelt's "fireside chats," and he would say in his best, deep Roosevelt voice, "I hate wor. Carol hates wor," and then he would put his finger in the air, change from his serious expression to delight, and add, "But … if there's going to be a wor, we want to be in the middle of it!" And he never shied from a "wor." It seemed to invigorate him.

Don was surprisingly funny. He was of quick wit and a dry humor, so it seemed to sneak up on people. He teased me incessantly. He tricked me into eating mountain oysters, which I swore I'd never do. In an elevator full of strangers, he would act as though we did not know each other, and he would come on to me with great zeal! If we were on the road, he might make up some wild story about why we were traveling together, and carry it on throughout our trip. He always made me feel that I was the only thing he saw through his eyes.

He was tender and quiet. He would take the babies and hold them close and walk silently with them—around the house, or down the street, or through the park. When my granddaughter Erin was only three months old and could not be comforted, Don took her for his "Grandpa walk." Suddenly, we noticed her crying had stopped and looked in to see him lying on the couch with his shirt off and Erin lying with her ear against his heart, her tiny hands clutching his bare chest, kneading his hair. They seemed to be lost in a silent duet of the soul. When he played with the children, he rarely spoke; he sat on the floor and drank from their teacups and held their dolls and made faces, and spoke a language only the children understood.

Don enjoyed the simple act of driving. He would put his left hand on the steering wheel and his right arm around me, and we would take off for anywhere, or nowhere. I called them his "whiplash trips" with a flick of my wrist and a "psst-choo." We would get into the car and drive someplace, eat dinner, stay the night, and drive straight back home—with no real purpose in mind. Don always said he was born a century too late and that he really belonged in the Wild West. For him, there was a romantic draw to a town he found on the map called Brownwood, Texas, and he fancied it might be a place he would like to live. One morning on Christmas Eve, we got into the car and drove toward Brownwood; we stayed overnight outside of Austin on Christmas Eve, lucky to find a room and a meal. On Christmas Day, we drove on to Brownwood; drove through the little town with a few run-down houses, a washer on every porch, and a donkey in every yard; and drove right on through. Don never even slowed down, and neither of us spoke a word as we looked at each other with a knowing smile. We left Texas, driving into a raging blizzard as we pressed home. We heard *Feliz Navidad* so many times on that trip that whenever we heard it again, we burst out laughing! Don never mentioned Brownwood, Texas, again, but that was certainly not our last "whiplash trip."

Through the hours we drove, we talked of hopes, dreams, and realistic goals for our life together. I wrote them down as we put them in order of their importance to us. We talked of what we would do if one of us died. We wrote down on the paper, "Die together." We fantasized about an oversized coffin where I would lay beside him just the way we did in bed—my head on his shoulder, my leg sprawled across his body, and we would sleep together for eternity.

In the end, we wrote down, "Talk to the kids about cremation."

We spent no time apart. When my best friend, Pamela Landis, asked me to meet her in Branson, Missouri, for a week, it was a major decision for Don and me. We finally decided that it was a wonderful opportunity for two old friends to be together again and I should go. I drove to Tulsa, where I met her plane, and we spent the week together, catching up on our lives. When I started the drive back home, Don called to tell me he was waiting for me in Pittsburgh, Kansas, about an eighth of the way back. We spent the night together there, and he followed me all the way home in his pickup, telling me he never wanted to be apart like that again.

Don didn't like Thanksgiving and Christmas, the same as he didn't like Valentine's Day. He would begin planning a way to bypass the dinners and family get-togethers early in November. We would take his whiplash trips or spend the holiday alone in a resort someplace where we would be the only guests on Christmas Day. Once we found ourselves in a tiny town on Christmas Day with not one restaurant open, not even a convenience store to buy a cold sandwich. We ate candy bars for Christmas dinner. Or we volunteered to prepare and serve Thanksgiving Dinner, with all the fixin's, at the Ronald McDonald House. Anything to break away from the traditional celebrations.

We tried to make our own family traditions: spaghetti for Thanksgiving dinner instead of turkey; the Christmas tree on the front porch instead of the parlor; the biggest party of the year an extravagant Halloween party. Don didn't do shopping, so his gifts were always most innovative. He wrote a series of short stories for me one year, each an analogy of the way he loved me. While we had Wear Purple, a friend of mine inherited her grandmother's wedding dress from the turn of the century and brought it in to show me. I was enchanted by the magnificent lace; it was the most beautiful thing I'd ever seen. Don saw my face that day and bought the wedding dress from my friend for me for Christmas. Everybody won; he didn't have to go shopping, and I got what I could have only dreamed of owning. The dress stands on an antique dress form in our home, and it has taken my breath away every day of my life.

After we closed the shop, we turned the space into an office where Don carried out his real estate and management business. I got my real estate license, and we worked together on every sale. I liked to find and show houses, and he liked to "close the deal" by writing the contract and procuring the financing. Between us, likening our business to fishing, we said, "Carol throws in the bait and catches them, and Don guts and cleans them!" I also started my own little oil and gas accounting business. The oil and gas business is a breed all its own, and I was acquainted with many of the "old boys," the first-generation oilmen in our city. As they retired, there was a need for accounting without the full office setting. I was known and trusted in the business. I would do their accounting on a weekly, monthly, or annual basis in my own office, which I shared with my husband. And so we settled into our office, enjoying everything we had accomplished together.

We lived quietly, but every day was a "trip"; we were never bored. Everything was on the periphery of our lives, with our relationship at the center. We loved our life together. We took in strays, both people and animals. I held the mice living in our shed, making sure all the grandkids got to see how cute they were. Soon after, I began to feel sick. Don laughed as he took me to the emergency room, because I just knew I had hantavirus. He rolled his eyes when I collected a beautiful live black widow spider for the children to see and preserved it perfectly in the freezer. He said, "Other children's grandmothers have turkeys in their freezer. Ours has a black widow spider!" We simply did things our own way.

Frank

And there was nephew Frank. Always, there was Frank. He was the one person Don allowed into our marriage. I first met him in a small pub with Don before we were married. Before our first meeting, anticipating my arrival, he told the waitress I was deaf in my right ear and she would have to compensate for me. Now, I love a good joke. But the waitress and I never knew what he had planned, and there was a kind of perverseness in that he was the only one to enjoy the joke. Don told me about it later; I was not offended, it just seemed pointless and for his entertainment only. From then on, I didn't trust Frank and always felt I was about to be on the receiving end of some cowardly prank. It was his way to do nothing in the open; he was like an amateur magician—he worked under a cloth so no one saw what he was doing until it was done, and then no one was sure how he did it. Don took Frank into his business, where I watched him misuse funds, indiscriminately charge personal items to the company accounts, and cause problems with every job he did. Don knew it, but chose to overlook it. Frank's presence in our home became a problem for me. He would just walk in when I was there alone, and finally Don put a stop to it when I found him asleep in our basement when I came home from work. When we visited Don's small hometown, I would hear talk of business lawsuits, and even federal charges, against him. I didn't understand any of it and didn't want to know about it. But I began to seriously question Don's judgment when it came to Frank.

Frank was as close to Don's children as if he were their brother. But there was something more to it. The family seemed to give Frank much more latitude than seemed reasonable. They seemed to hide his faults, excuse his indiscretions, and overlook his apparent crimes. No matter what he did, the family would not hold Frank accountable for his actions. Don would not make him quit taking from his company or pay him back; he would not even bring it to his attention! He was surrounded by enablers who led him to believe he was entitled to whatever he desired. I began to call Frank the family's "Sacred Cow." Their unconditional support of him was that irrational.

Frank was J.R.'s only son, raised as a cattle buyer. J.R. died before I met Don. Upon his father's death, Frank had been expected to take over the family ranch—which did not fit into his life's plan. Frank's mother, Iona, was a sweet little farm lady, who by the time I met her was in very poor health. In our visits to Iona's Oklahoma home, conversation was always about Frank and the trouble he was in. I overheard enough to be really concerned about his morality. In quiet voices, Iona and Don talked about large amounts of money that she needed and that Frank would not repay. And then he quit responding to her phone calls and refused to see her or communicate with her. After complications with surgery, Iona spent months in an Oklahoma hospital and then a rehabilitation center. Don and I spent nearly every weekend at the hospital with her. She called for Frank, but he would not come. He made one short visit to her bedside when she thought she was dying, but that was the last. How a man treats his mother is the most telling of traits. I had no use for him and could not understand how his family could overlook such actions.

When Iona began to recover, she came to our home for Thanksgiving, and we all met for the evening at Carla's home. Iona was excited that Frank was going to be there; she longed to just have a conversation with her son. Frank dominated the evening with talk about his active life and how he helped acquaintances make a major move across country, aiding them because the wife had been diagnosed with multiple sclerosis. Iona's presence was ignored completely, and she left the room in her wheelchair in tears. I followed her; the two of us seemed to be the only two who felt the slap in the face to a loving mother. She was hurt that he would give so much of himself to help a stranger, and brag about it, but not seem to care that his own mother was infirm and needed him. Of all of Frank's sins, this was the one for which I held him most accountable.

Don was not willing to deal with Frank. He always saw what he was doing, but he skipped over his actions like a blip on a screen. Don and I had a strong marriage, and we did not argue or fight. We did disagree, and most of our disagreements were over Frank. He always made me think of "Pigpen" in the Peanuts cartoon. Everywhere he went, chaos followed him like Pigpen's filth. He was unpredictable and disruptive, and he brought confusion to every encounter. He was suggestive and offensive, and he lied about everything, even about things that didn't matter to anyone. Chaos was his drug of choice. Over the years, we experienced so many ridiculous situations with Frank that I came to avoid him as much as I could. For a time, he worked for Larry, Don's son-in-law, in the service department of a car dealership. Of course, we always took our vehicles there for service, until I overheard him tell how when women brought their cars in and tried to describe the problem, he would ask them to "make the noise" they were hearing, and then would laugh and make fun of them after they left. I quit taking my car in at all; I left that party to Don. But because Frank was the family Sacred Cow, it was difficult avoiding Frank. Many times, I escaped from his presence for Don to find me crying over my frustration and disappointment that Don would not deal with Frank. Nothing ever changed, and finally I accepted that this was the family I married into, and this part of it had to be separate from me.

Both Don and I seemed to grow more content and happy with every year we were married. We had our "Frank moments" but I didn't have to live with him, so they were always a passing thing, and I left him entirely to Don.

I often felt too happy! As though there would be a price to pay for this happiness, I sometimes wondered when the other shoe was going to drop, but as the years went on, the shoes seemed to be firmly on our feet.

The Quarry, 1998

My longtime employer, Mr. Roberts, had spent the last decade of his life buying pasture land in the coveted Kansas Flint Hills. It was his hobby. In all, he bought 3,000 acres of prime Flint Hills pasture land and, along with it, an old abandoned rock quarry that was now a beautiful rock-lined lake. There was a cabin on the property, and the fish were so plentiful that at times they jumped out of the water onto the dock! Our family had free run of the Quarry for the years Mr. Roberts owned it. I dealt personally with all of the ranchers and farmers around the Roberts land, managing the properties and taking care of all the business. Mr. Roberts had an impeccable reputation, which I was fortunate enough to inherit from him. After Mr. Roberts's death, Don and I were given the opportunity to buy any of his acreage we wanted, and we bought the Quarry and the surrounding quarter section. We planned to build a home someday on the property and began to landscape, build docks, and upgrade the property. Don loved the part that reminded him of his farm roots. He loved to get on the tractor and mow, row after row, around and around. We had two tractors, and sometimes I would mow with one, and sometimes I would ride on Don's tractor behind him, like one would ride double on a horse. I would sing *Happy Trails* in his ear as we laughed at ourselves being Roy Rogers and Dale Evans, watching the sun go down on our beautiful Flint Hills pastures.

We spent every spare minute landscaping, building with the natural stones from the quarry, which seemed to grow out of the earth like plants. When we hauled one away for our projects, another emerged in its place. I would look up from where I was setting the natural stones into steps to see Don on his old grey and red Ford tractor, pulling a huge stone he'd found behind with a chain. I would stop and laugh as I watched him come toward me, grinning, with his precious bounty. When we were too tired to pick up another stone, I would dive into the cool waters of the quarry, while Don sat quietly in the boat with his fishing pole in the water, and we would end our day together.

The Quarry became our party place. Everyone we knew looked forward to going out with us for the day, or to one of our large parties. Our grandchildren all caught their first fish there. The lake was clean; we had a playground for the children with a sand pile, slide, and swings. We had paddleboats, fishing boats, tire swings over the water, a swimming dock with a slide, hay wagons, and an abandoned "spook" house out in the pasture. We had summer swimming parties, barn dances, live bands, Fourth of July fireworks, Halloween hayrides, scavenger hunts, bonfires, and elaborate haunted houses. We had theme parties like a fifties, sixties, and seventies party, where I was Mousketeer Annette and Don was Moondoggie; there was an abundance of poodle skirts, polyester suits, and go-go boots. Don and I became well-known for our great family parties. Our parties were planned for the children as well as the adults, and the Quarry was a place the kids could safely spend the day as children might have a hundred years ago. We set up music to match the theme of the party at one end of the Quarry, which could be heard to the other end. We danced to *Monster Mash* at Halloween, *Born in the USA* on the Fourth of July, and *Jeremiah Was a Bullfrog* in late summer. We smoked brisket all day until the wonderful aroma couldn't be ignored anymore. We had pie throws and Hula-hoop contests. We set up a dance floor under the stars, and everyone danced late into the dark. Many of our family and guests had never danced before, but they made up their own dances and played like children along with the music until we were all exhausted. One guest was overheard saying, "No matter how we might try, there will never be another night as magical as this." Friends and family brought out their campers and tents, and my brother even put up his authentic Indian teepee from time to time to spend a week on the prairie.

Always looking for something different to add to the Quarry, I bought a sailboat at a local yard sale. On the Quarry water, there just wasn't enough wind to sail it. That sailboat was about the only thing I ever saw Don not able to master. He kept trying, but developed what I thought was a hilarious hatred for it. So, instead of sailing, we would sit in the boat, just Don and me, feet in the water, listening to the summer sounds of cicadas and tree frogs in an otherwise perfectly still world. We would sit through the black night on the banks of the Quarry, holding hands, and watch meteor showers. It was our place of peace.

Meanwhile ...

Frank needed a place to live. We needed a caretaker, and the little shack suited him just fine. So Frank lived at the Quarry until he took up residency in the El Dorado Correctional Facility.

In the fall of 1997, Frank's trial was held in the county courthouse. Frank had made another cattle deal. In the end, again, there were no cattle, and he could not account for the $156,000 he was paid for them. Sensitive as I was to his feelings, I reminded him that a hundred years ago he would have been hung for cattle rustling! He had no defense. Don and I and Carla, Don's daughter, attended the trial, and Don was called to the stand as the only defense witness—a character reference. I watched Don struggle to defend Frank's character, but he could not. It was a sad day; I had never seen Don embarrassed over anything before, but that day he was humiliated because he could think of nothing to say and he knew he sounded ridiculous. Frank was sentenced to a year in prison and ordered to make restitution, which of course he could not do.

This situation was ominously like the Wyoming cattle failure for which Don accepted full responsibility, but Don refused to speak about it with me. We all suspected that somewhere on the Quarry grounds there was a hole containing $156,000.

The family, including Don, gathered around Frank and treated his crime as though it were a joke. I was furious with Frank for sullying our name in the community, where our last name, which I shared with him and with Don, was known and associated with Mr. Robert's name. This was the last straw for me with him. It seemed no one was willing to hold him accountable for his actions except me. In effect, I drew a line in the sand and stood alone against Frank. He had a friend live at the Quarry for the year he was in prison to secure his return to it when he got out. When he returned, the games resumed in full force. Iona, Frank's mother, told me, "You took his playmate away," and Frank seemed determined to punish me for that and come between Don and me any way he could.

The Descent Begins

One morning in September of 2000, Don got out of bed and walked right into the wall. He had lost his equilibrium, was confused, and couldn't seem to get his body to follow his orders. We thought that he must have had a small stroke. He recovered fairly quickly, or at least it appeared that he did. Of course we immediately saw his doctor, who began clinical testing, but there was no indication from the exhaustive tests that anything was wrong. Don used his great will to regain his balance and forced himself to recover. For months, he would stand on one leg while shaving to improve his balance; he would run backwards; he pushed himself as though he was defying impairment.

That day in September was the beginning of his journey to Purgatory.

As time went on, we saw other signs of TIAs (small strokes). Don was, unlike me, one of those people who loved exercise, took vitamins, and ate right. He jogged several miles every morning—until it became too exhausting and he worried that he was pushing himself too hard. He regretted it when he had to stop. His decline was so subtle that we could put nothing together. He began to feel unwell; his stomach was always upset; sometimes the nausea was extreme and debilitating. Don was obviously ill, but the doctors could find no cause. So, life went on, with good days and bad days, but Don tried to ignore his illness as much as he could.

Memorial Day of 2004, we planned a day of celebrating with the whole family at the Quarry. Frank knew we were all coming out, but we found the grass high and unmowed and the property in unkempt condition; Frank was nowhere to be found. He had removed the batteries from the tractor and boat, parked the equipment to block roads, and stored away the lawn furniture to make it as difficult as he possibly could for us. He had left the Quarry in that state on that Memorial Day, but Don went right to work, charging batteries and moving the equipment. He spent the whole day mowing around the Quarry. He was ill when the day started and was exhausted by the time we left the Quarry that day; he could hardly function. Not knowing I was foretelling the future, I told Don, "I will never go there again as long as Frank lives there." I wasn't threatening my husband, because I already knew after fourteen years of marriage that when it came to taking sides between Frank and me, the family would *always* side with Frank, even my husband. It was simply a decision I made for myself. That was the last time either of us ever went to the Quarry.

By the summer of 2004, Don's mystery illness was worsening. He rarely felt like going to the office. He began to feel threatened and afraid of people and situations. He was uncomfortable in public and unsure of himself in any situation. He didn't want to go out of the house, and he didn't want me to go out either.

We had moved into a new house in late 2002. We had lovely neighbors, but since we had lived in our house only a short time, we had only a "waving" relationship. In the spring of 2004, the woman next door died of cancer. That was when I began to see that Don was becoming paranoid and unreasonable in his thoughts. He accused me of having an affair with the poor man who had just lost his wife, and nothing I could say would relieve him of this thought. I spent the whole summer peeking around corners before going into the yard, ignoring even the neighborly waves. Don finally gave that accusation up, but then out of the blue, he said he'd been watching me with the man across the street. First with one neighbor, then with the other, then with men I had never met. He was obviously tortured by his thoughts but I couldn't find enough ways to reassure him. He began to say, almost in a panic, that he wanted to get married and did not realize that we had been married for fourteen years.

By the first of July, every time I left the house for work, Don panicked, and his panic transferred to me. I began to have sudden, painful headaches followed by faintness. I thought this must be what a stroke felt like. As I left for work one morning, I said to myself, "If it happens this morning, I am going straight to the doctor's office," and in an hour I was being examined.

The doctor explained to me that my symptoms indicated stress rather than a stroke; after I explained what was going on at home, he asked to see Don. After examining and testing him, he sent him directly to a cardiologist. Don's heart catheterization showed significant problems. Open heart surgery was scheduled for the following week. However, the next day, Don began to feel as though he was having a heart attack. We called the heart hospital and raced there, where they waited for him with a gurney. On July 9, 2004, Don had emergency quintuple by-pass heart surgery. The doctors said that when he had the surgery, Don was within hours of having a massive heart attack. In the heart hospital, they go about this surgery as though it's nothing, just routine and simple. They said Don came through the surgery just fine and had no heart damage. One of his main arteries was 100 percent clogged, but we learned that the body has the amazing ability to restructure itself. Because he had exercised and kept his body in shape, new smaller veins had developed to carry the blood around the useless artery, which prevented damage to the heart. As a family, we rejoiced that Don was given back to us whole.

So, we went home from the hospital with a red heart-shaped pillow as a memento, anxious for Don's recovery and to get back to the life we had been missing for several years now. We were so happy to have found the answer that would end Don's illness. But nothing stands alone in this life, and behind the scenes what was happening was both a blessing and horrifying.

Matters of the Heart

I was never alone at the heart hospital. All six of our children were there with us as much as they could be, taking turns sitting with me or Don. Most of the time, we were all sitting in the little side room together, waiting for the opportunity to see Don, who was in ICU. My son Rob and I have always been close. Love was a tangible thing in our home, as it was just natural to touch, hug, or kiss whenever we passed by each other. The outward expression of my love with Don was equally as natural, but I had not seen that warmth between Don and his children. Apparently, Don's children had not been raised to feel comfortable showing affection outwardly, but the warmth they saw between us drew them. They wanted what they saw between my son and me. The girls asked me how they could express their love as Rob and I did. It was obvious that they felt they had missed this relationship with their father. They had a genuine hunger and need for the physical expression of their love to and from their dad. So, we talked, we hugged, and we expressed our appreciation for one another. It touched me greatly when Carla said to me, "I am so thankful that Dad has you." When we returned home, I wrote in my journal:

> *Our six kids are wonderful. I feel now like I have a new family. We had to join together in our love for*

Don to get him through this, and we did. None of us alone, but like arms and legs working together to make something happen. We became one body—one family.

But while our family was bonding and finding love in the waiting room, in the operating room, Don was enduring what no one should have to remember. But he remembered it all vividly. I can only imagine from the long, red scar from his neck to his navel, how ravaged his body was. His bones were sawed in two, and his heart was removed. Is this not death? What happens to the id, the ego, the self, while one's heart has stopped beating? Where does the soul go while the body is in suspended animation? During the surgery, while they held his heart in their hands, he could hear a conversation between the doctors, word for word, trying to decide what to do about the complications they saw. He remembered the room and the sights during the surgery itself. The anesthesia had produced detachment, not unconsciousness. Don told of seeing the huge light above the operating table, he described the equipment for the surgery, and as the cardiologist held Don's heart in his hands, he heard the cardiologist say to his associate, "Well, got any ideas?"

What I saw when I was allowed to be with him after the surgery was horrifying: the huge drain tube protruding from his abdomen; tubes for medicine; tubes for monitoring; the intubation of his throat—which he prematurely and violently pulled out of his own body. He was obviously not in control of his mind. He had a wild look in his eyes, a look of panic, and I began to panic myself because there was nothing I could do to relieve him of his imaginings. He insisted that I must get him out of that place, *now*. He told me a story of sabotage. He was sure that he was in a place where his death was being plotted. He said if I did not get him out, they were going to kill him. When I tried to explain that it was impossible, that all of the tubes and connections were there to keep him alive, he only became more angry and insistent. He said if I didn't help him, our marriage was over; that he couldn't love me any more. Although I knew this must be the drugs, still I was confused, desperate, and terrified. There was nothing I could say to him that would make him stop this madness. I had to leave him alone in his own terror while I sat on the hallway floor and wept in mine. This new man, who was a stranger to me, came to live with us and never left.

All the next day, he hallucinated about surreal and nightmarish situations from which he begged—demanded—I rescue him. At dusk, he was moved out of the ICU, and I was told to go home and sleep. I did go home, but although I was exhausted, I couldn't settle down in my bed alone. I turned on the television and stared blindly at the screen, trying to escape the world to which I knew I would have to return. At 2:30 am, the phone woke me out of sleep and paralyzed me with fear. The caller said that Don was combative and uncontrollable, and asked if I could come and try to calm him down. When I arrived, there were two large male nurses in his room. Don was holding them at bay, and they could not control him. When I walked into the room, Don was muttering to himself and was going through the motions of physically fighting off some imaginary antagonist. At first, he was so lost in his delusion that he didn't seem to know me. But as I talked to him, he calmed down. I took him down the hall in a wheelchair, and when we came back to his room, I crawled into the little hospital bed with him and told him I would stay with him and hold him in my arms. He was like a child having a terrible nightmare. Clinging to each other, we slept the few hours before dawn. In the morning, he not only remembered the whole scenario of the night before, he had a very detailed, elaborate story to tell about being taken to the basement of a warehouse and held captive. He had to outwit them to escape, and that is what he was doing when I came—carrying out his plan to escape. Not only did he stick to his story, he actually believed it happened.

After surgery, Don's stay in the hospital was four days. The whole time, he hallucinated and had severe anxiety attacks. The doctor told me the hallucinations and episodes of psychosis—effects of the surgery—could last as long as six weeks, maybe more. I had no idea how we were going to integrate hallucinations, delusions, and psychosis into our lives, but clung to the doctor's words that they would end.

The first few months, we expected illness, but we also expected every day to be better than the last. We waited for the better. Physically, Don healed quickly, and the cardiologist's reports were right on target. He returned to his work. We resumed our social life. The earliest symptoms that something else was wrong was that he quit reading; he became much more dependent on me to do everyday things; he could not play cards, or games of any kind, at which he always used to blow us all away. He couldn't count or match up dominoes. But he would laugh and act as though he was teasing, and I would wonder why he wasn't trying. He had always been competitive in everything, saying, "Show me someone who says they don't care if they win, and I'll show you a loser" (that would be me).

Soon, his depression turned to anxiety, to debilitating nausea, and to paranoia. He began making major financial mistakes in his business, and the girls in the office were concerned for Don and for the future of the business. He lost his grip on how to run his company, losing the ability to even use the phone. Eventually, he became unable to even go to the office or anyplace else outside the house. He seemed to be paralyzed with fear and anxiety.

Don said throughout the whole experience that he felt no pain at all in his body. But it was obvious that his spirit was greatly suffering. He was different. He didn't understand the changes in himself, and he didn't know this man who was living in his body. He couldn't think in the same way, respond in the same way, and he became a blur of his former self—unrecognizable to him. He could not recover his sense of self. He was experiencing a great sense of loss. It seemed that with the surgery and the anesthesia, Don's self had fragmented as he watched the invasion of his body from above, but all of the pieces of himself were never able to reconnect as his heart began to beat again. He felt a vulnerability and lack of self-confidence that left him confused and lost. I thought of "Star Trek," when someone commanded, "Beam me up, Scotty," and the person fragmented and disappeared to find himself reappearing on a different planet. What if something went wrong and the parts didn't realign the same?

Who would he be? Don seemed to feel he had awakened on another planet, missing the essential parts of his personality.

One day while waiting in a doctor's office with Don and Dale, I said to Dale, "Don lies to the doctors. He will not tell them what is going on," to which he replied, "I do that, too! I make a game of it!" I guess I was supposed to laugh with him, but I just stared at him in disbelief. Dr. House is right: Everyone lies. I have learned that doctors do not allow the time it takes to get the truth from a patient. Our medical care is totally up to us; we must know our symptoms and we must insist that the doctors listen to us. We have to do our homework and ask the right questions.

In the doctor's office, Don would distract his physician with talk of fishing or the days when they played basketball together. The doctor, whom Don had known for a long time, would slap him on the back and say, "He looks great to me!" and walk out. I was just dumbfounded, because Don had not told the doctor anything that was going on, and I was given virtually no chance to speak. The next time, when the back-slapping came, I stood between the doctor and the door and said, "The man cannot function!" Once the doctor was forced to hear what was really going on with Don, he began to treat him.

Thus began a long list of trial-and-error drugs: Remron, Xanax, Buspar, Prozac, Paxil, Lexapro, Zoloft, Effexor, Cymbalta, and Seroquel, and an extensive parade of doctors. We saw a psychiatrist, a psychologist, a neurologist, an optometrist; we saw a stomach doctor, a colon doctor, a foot doctor; we had MRIs, sonograms, EEGs.

The doctors thought he wasn't getting enough oxygen to his brain and was sleep deprived. So we went through the sleep clinic … twice. The first overnight stay, they called me at 3:00 am to pick Don up because he was having panic attacks and was not able to go to sleep, so the tests were not completed. The second time, I was asked to stay with him overnight, and with me beside him, he slept. He was diagnosed with severe sleep apnea, which is interruption or cessation of breathing during sleep, causing sleep deprivation (it can even lead to death). This diagnosis was no surprise to me, as most nights were a mixture of watching Don, almost in a panic, waiting for him to take a breath or being nearly knocked out of bed by violent awakenings as he gasped for a breath. The treatment was wearing a C-PAP machine during the night, which is a mask with a hose connected to a humidifier. It was very intrusive and confining, so Don would not use it, and his sleep simply became more violent every night.

His symptoms were vast, and there was a different doctor for each one. Visiting each new doctor presented its own set of problems. The first psychologist was on the third floor of a building. When the elevator opened, Don refused to get on and ran out of the building. In the next psychologist's office, he decided he did not want to take the tests and refused, trying to flee the office like a child. This would not be the last time I was left standing in a doctor's office alone without the patient.

Don had always had a measure of claustrophobia, but it increased as his paranoia worsened. He was not only anxious about being in a small space, he believed that he was the target of persecution and that what was happening to him was an intentional assault or attack on him. When Don was scheduled for an MRI, we had to find an open MRI, and even then, he was full of anxiety. Getting him into a hospital gown was a challenge, as he was so paranoid that he began to imagine the doctors, nurses, and I were his enemy. The MRI was difficult for Don, and for me, as it was my job to keep him calm and still through it. When he was ready to get dressed, he had a catastrophic reaction, which happens when the person loses all coping skills and becomes uncontrollable, somewhat like a six-foot, two hundred-pound child throwing a fit. He refused to go into the room to get out of the gown and back into his street clothes. When I could not get him to calm down, it was decided I would take him home as he was. It was late winter and it was cold and wet outside, as the snow was melting. I brought the car to the door, driving on the sidewalk, and put him in, barefoot, with only a hospital gown on. He was very angry with me for letting this happen to him. Everything was my fault. I became the enemy. Life was getting more complicated with every day.

He was diagnosed in the spring of 2005 with mild cognitive impairment, an illness affecting the area of the brain that has to do with cognitive abilities such as decision making; it is a precursor to Alzheimer's. That didn't sound so bad. Denny Crane has that, and he still manages "Boston Legal"! Denny Crane calls it "mad cow." But unlike Denny Crane, Don's cognitive abilities were rapidly declining. And this was no laughing matter. The cognitive drugs began ... Aricept and Exelon.

2006

By the end of 2005, Don was not able to go into the office. For the last year, he had been ill, and although he had been at the office almost every day, apparently he was not functioning well. Don's secretary had been doing her best to keep the company going and cover for him, but the situation became overwhelming. She gave notice that she was leaving January 1, 2006. I went in over the holiday to look at the books. There had been no reconciliations done, Don was not keeping bank registers, and the bank account was in arrears by $10,000! I found that over the last few years, Don had allowed several tenants to slide on rent, and the company was thousands of dollars in arrears to property owners. Security deposits had been used as working capital. Don had loaned two different tenants large amounts of money, with little hope of it being repaid. He had allowed a contractor to draw on a client's maintenance account without ever doing the work. He had cosigned on a loan for a tenant who, of course, never made a payment himself on the loan before disappearing.

    I always considered myself a problem solver, but I wasn't sure there was a solution to these problems. For two weeks, I hardly slept as I meditated and prayed for wisdom to fix this mess. I couldn't just close the company … too much money was unaccounted for. And I wanted to keep it alive because Don talked constantly about getting back to the office. I saw it as his motivation for getting better, and I still believed he could get better. I moved myself into the office and tried to reorganize the business so we could recover. With Don at home, my own business to keep up with, the real estate company (for which I was the closest thing to a broker now), I had little patience for the all-consuming management company, which was fast becoming a monster that had to be fed at the expense of everything else. I would have let it die if I could have, but the act of cleaning up the mess would have been far more devastating than keeping it alive.

This was not my "wor." I don't have the temperament to interact with tenants who feel entitled and landlords who, for a few dollars a month, want you to cater to their every need. I would just as soon say to a tenant, "There are plenty of other houses in town ... go find one!" or tell a landlord, "Just see if you can find some other idiot to do all you want done for what Don charged!" I longed for my little cubbyhole with my numbers, which always added up and never changed. I missed my classical music ... and my peace. I missed my best friend, with whom I shared everything and who always knew what to do. I prayed for God to give me divine guidance, as I was fresh out of anything that resembled wisdom.

Don's daughter, Carla, knew we were in a crisis with the business, and she wanted to help her father. All the children offered to do whatever they could, but this was a day-time business and they all had their own jobs and families to attend to. Carla offered to work at the business part time, which would help me reorganize, catch up, and keep things going. She started, but after less than a month, she disappeared. She was working on projects after hours or at home, so I didn't realize she had quit until it became obvious that the work hadn't been done. She probably thought it was hopeless, to which I would not have disagreed at all. I called her and asked if she had lost interest, and she said it just wasn't working out for her. There wasn't much to argue with. I picked up her projects and went on. I didn't have time to despair, but I prayed for help.

One day, a young man named Chuck walked into the office. Although he was well acquainted with our business, I had been out of the office on a regular basis for so long I didn't know who he was.

He had an appliance repair business and was doing much of the maintenance work for the company. He was very capable, and he had a way of handling people, much like Don. Like a miracle, each time I would think, "I need Chuck," he would walk in the door. I didn't know what the plan was, but I knew there was a divine purpose in Chuck being there at that time. And as often is God's way, Chuck was in a place where our situation was about to be his miracle as well.

At the Quarry, Frank continued to keep visitors out, and the grounds began to deteriorate. He had an ever-growing number of dogs and cats living in the house, but he was rarely at the shack anymore. We called it the most expensive doghouse in Kansas! There were problems between my family members, who were invited to use the Quarry, and Frank (e.g., upon being notified they were coming, he would chain the gates closed). It became too troublesome for anyone other than Don's children to use the Quarry, so it got little use. In the meantime, Don's health continued to fail.

In the early spring of 2006, I received a call from the electric company saying all other services had been cut off at the Quarry for nonpayment, and if there was no longer anyone living there, they were also going to turn off electrical service. This was pretty definite evidence that Frank was no longer staying there. Don and I began talking to the kids to see if anyone had any interest in us keeping the Quarry. We thought we should sell it, since no one was able to enjoy it, and unattended, it was a great liability. Word got to Frank that we were talking to the kids about selling the Quarry. One morning in late spring, on a rare occasion that Don was in the office with me, Frank walked in and announced that we could not sell it unless we sold it to him, and for the same price we paid. The trauma of this outburst triggered Don's anxiety and paranoia, and he stood rigid, pale, and frightened. Not me! I finally had my chance to speak my mind, to tell Frank how little I thought of him and his games that hurt other people. I ordered him out of our office in terms that I admit were not worthy of his Sacred Cow status.

By Memorial Day 2006, Don and I sought legal advice from our attorney. Frank, claiming that he still lived at the Quarry, had the sympathy of Don's children. James and Doug, being attorneys, decided they could help settle this amicably and began to intervene; Doug took the position of neutral mediator and negotiated a sales contract. James took the position of representing Frank. Don and I were not unhappy to leave everything as it was and just not think about it, but the family's involvement took it to the next level. We didn't care if Frank bought the Quarry; however, he would have to pay the fair market value, and he did not have the money to do so. The family attorneys did not seem to understand that Frank could not afford such a purchase and pursued with lengthy negotiations.

There were much more important things going on in our lives than to spend our time and emotions on Frank. And Don had been so traumatized by the day in the office (probably more by his own inability to stand up to him than by Frank himself) that he not only wanted him out of our lives, but he was frightened of him. I was startled when Don told our attorney that he believed Frank was capable of physically harming us. I could not imagine Frank as anything but a coward, but Don said he had seen him become violent and knew what he was capable of. One of Frank's well-known traits was his penchant for revenge. He would make an intricate game of plotting revenge when he felt offended. I actually thought it was only mind games, which he never carried out. Don disagreed. During the family negotiations for the Quarry, the phone rang about nine one evening. Don answered the phone, and I could tell from his demeanor that he was extremely uncomfortable with the call. He concluded the call with "Don't ever call here again" in a deep monotone, and he was visibly upset. He said it was Frank calling from some bar, and he had threatened him, using language that frightened him. Don was afraid to go to sleep that night and sat up in bed watching the door for as long as he could. From that time forward, Don's paranoia increased, and his delusions and hallucinations became more threatening and violent, and very dark.

Offers were bantered back and forth, sometimes coming from us, sometimes coming from Frank and James. Ultimately, Frank didn't have any money to buy the Quarry, and by July all the talk of his buying it was forgotten. So life went on … Frank at the Quarry, and Don and I fighting our own battle for his life. At some point, we intended to sell the Quarry, but there was no time or energy to think about that now. Don's health was foremost on our list of priorities.

But this was not the last we were going to hear from Frank. His past crimes would not be his last. He would later prove to be terrifyingly vengeful by writing many long, vile, disgusting letters to me with veiled threats, satisfying his taste for revenge with unthinkable accusations.

In the meantime, Kate, Carla, and I worked together to get the diagnosis and treatment needed for their dad. I don't throw in the towel easily, and on this level, I was not alone. We were determined to research, by trial and error, to find the right doctors and get whatever drugs would make Don well. Kate is somewhat educated in psychiatric drugs, and Carla worked for a hospital, where she did medical and pharmaceutical research. Each of us had come up with a new disease we wanted him tested for, or a new doctor he should see. I often said he had been to every kind of doctor except a gynecologist, and that was next! Every doctor ordered all new tests—and the same old ones over and over again.

But we still had few answers, and Don was getting worse every day. By September of 2006, Kate made an appointment with a geriatrics specialist. A barrage of blood tests began, and we found that Don was B-12 depleted. The normal number is around 600, and Don was at 150. Who knew that vitamin B-12 was so important? B-12 is what keeps the nervous system healthy. The symptoms of a B-12 deficiency range from reduced cognitive function to dementia and neurological changes such as numbness or tingling, depression, inability to maintain balance, and poor memory. Because he had all of these symptoms, we thought we finally had a fixable answer. I took him directly to begin B-12 shots that very day. When he got the first shot, we were warned that the body can store B-12 for up to a year, but if the deprivation goes longer than that, the brain damage could be irreversible. Like Scarlett O'Hara, we wouldn't think about that today.

Don's children all seemed to follow in their father's physical footsteps. They all had bouts with panic attacks, depression, ADD, and other medical problems that they seemed to have inherited from their father's side of the family—especially Carla and Doug. We immediately let the kids know that they should be checked for B-12 deficiency. Doug's levels particularly put him at risk, and he began treatment. Don and I said that if this was all about saving just one of the kids, then it was worth it for him to have gone through this.

July 30, 2006

It is after noon, and Don is still asleep. So, this may be what he does with his day while I'm away. I try to take stock of his condition—at times I think his mind is gone; he cannot function. But I close the door to our home and he is the same as he always was with me. Family asks how I am doing, and I honestly don't feel anything is wrong when Don and I are alone. He likes it that way. Us alone. He will do about anything to keep me alone with him. Of course, all of it—and having to do business for us both—wears me down. And sometimes I ask myself—why are you not afraid? Or crazy? Or worried about how things may be? And I don't know the answers. Don is still Don to me. (from my journal)

After the first round of B-12 treatments, we thought Don seemed better, and we were thankful for any improvement, or hope. While researching B-12 deficiency, I came across an article that said that anesthetics used for surgery can spontaneously deplete the body of B-12. The article said that usually B-12 is administered before or after surgery to build up the supply. I requested Don's records and found that he had not been given B-12, although his numbers were dangerously low every time they were taken at the hospital. All indications to me were that Don had experienced spontaneous depletion of B-12 during his heart surgery, and in actuality, he had been depleted since 2004, resulting in irreversible brain damage.

The last trip Don and I made together was in September 2006; we went to Don's fifty-fifth high school class reunion. He had made no effort to stay in contact with his classmates, and the word *reunion* was not dear to either of us. But a few of his old friends had been diligent about sending Don Christmas cards and making occasional calls throughout the decades. Don still had a couple of sisters-in-law in his little home town, so it wasn't really so difficult to stay in touch with the few who came out of that small town.

When the invitation to the reunion came, he threw it away. But as the time drew nearer, he began to receive notes and calls from his classmates, wanting him especially to come. I was impressed at their persistence and their sincere desire to see Don after so many years. Not only did I encourage him to go, I put him in the car on a beautiful September morning and drove him there, ignoring his protests.

Everyone was in the town square. It was like going back a hundred years, in that little town just across the border in Oklahoma. Food was being cooked and served in the streets, the smell of barbeque was enticing, music was playing, and children were enjoying rides in wagons pulled by donkeys or goats. The day had a touch of fall and was perfect for being outside. Children played in the streets, and in the open pavilion, little groups were forming as classmates arrived and became reacquainted. As soon as we made our way into the square, it seemed the word was passed, and Don's friends from long ago came to find him. Six of his classmates were there (a few had passed away). They caught him up in talk of school days and stories, and I just watched from a short distance as he enjoyed the attention. There was to be an exhibition basketball game in the old auditorium, where he had once been a star, and he was most anxious for that; in fact, he had it in his mind he would be playing that day. He went into the gym with his friends and they made him feel like a star again. It was such a pleasure for me to see him enjoy his friends and the whole day so much.

But he was obviously disoriented at times, and he stumbled a lot. We had wanted to keep his condition close to the vest, but it was no secret that he was ill. He looked hale and very handsome, and young for his age, but there was that lost look in his eyes and almost a mask on his face. He tired early, and we left in the afternoon. As I drove away on the dirt road with the red dust flying behind us, I asked him if he had a good time. He said yes, he had. "Did you remember all of your classmates?" "I have *no* idea who those people were, not one!" he answered. And we both laughed.

In October, Don began having more anxiety, paranoia, and panic attacks. One day, he thought he was having a heart attack, so we spent the next three days in the heart hospital; they did another cath and found his heart doing sufficiently well. Again, he had delusions while there, and the paranoia was intolerable. I slept beside him in the hospital all three nights, and yet he would awaken and forget that I was there and run down the hall looking for me. The children were there as before, staying long hours to be there for him. There was no doubt my husband was loved.

This visit to the hospital seemed to usher in a new phase: constant and unbelievably real hallucinations. He would wake in the night and see people—whom he could identify, but not someone he'd ever known—sitting in the chair beside the bed, just watching him. One night, he saw a man and woman in the room. The man held a gun pointed at him. Don heard the woman order the man to put the gun down. It was incomprehensible to me that these hallucinations were so real that he heard their voices. He began waking me in the night, hitting me and grabbing at what he thought was a gun I held. He would see people in the darkness of the hallway; he would see guns lying around; and possibly most disturbing, he would see the mirror on the armoire across from our bed airing pornography. He said, "How do they do that? Broadcast that kind of stuff over a mirror?" All rational thinking seemed to be gone at these times, and no amount of reasoning or explaining made any sense to him. I had to cover the mirror with a drape for him to go to sleep from that time on.

Why pornography? Here was a man who never found that interesting, and never indulged in such things. He thought it degrading. Why would that be what he saw in his psychosis?

He would see animals in our bed. Sometimes he would wake, trying to get them to stop chewing on his feet. He would look out the windows, any time of day or night, and see bears, wild dogs, or people looking in. He seemed undaunted by any of these visions, which I could not understand. They frightened me just to hear about them. I am a very spiritual person. I was raised Pentecostal, attended seminary, and was a teacher of doctrines in our church; I believed! I believe in a spiritual world, and I believe in God's intervention in our lives, and therefore, I believe in an evil counterpart to God. I wanted to know to which world these invaders belonged. I wanted Don to ask them who they were, where they came from, and why they visited him. I wanted him to talk to them: maybe they were real, and I was the only one who could not see them. I was trying to make sense of something that was senseless. But he wasn't afraid of them, or interested. They left when he willed them to, and he seemed to have no desire to discuss anything with them.

I was working at a client's office across town one morning when Don called me and said, "The people are here to start the renovation on the house." *Renovation?* He just wanted to let me know they were starting in the bedroom. I asked him if there was someone in charge that I could talk to, and he said there was a woman who was the contractor. I asked him if I could speak to her, thinking he would say, "Ha! There's no one here," but he said yes, he would take the phone to her. I heard him walk, phone in hand, across the house and into the bedroom, and I heard him say in his business voice, "Excuse me. My wife would like to speak to you" and then there was silence for a few seconds. Then he said into the phone to me, "She asked if she could talk to you later."

It is one of those moments when it takes awhile to digest what has just happened. I told him to sit down and wait … I would be home in twenty minutes. I wasn't sure what I was going to find when I got home: walls painted red, or knocked out? When I got home, he was calm and had decided that it was all a hallucination. To him, it was all over with! Not so for me! How real would a hallucination have to be for him to actually hand the phone to someone who wasn't really there? How does it happen that something that is not there is that real? How is it that he is calm?

Another day, he called me and said, with obvious desperation in his voice, that he was very tired, but he could not sit down because other people were taking all the chairs. He said there was a poker game going on in our living room, and there were so many people that he couldn't find a place for himself; in fact, he was lucky to even be able to use the phone. He said he was going outside to walk because he couldn't stand it anymore. I asked him who was there, and he said, "There are some famous people and a lot of other people I don't know." Again, I told him not to go out, but to try to find a place to rest, and I would be home in twenty minutes.

I walked in to find him calmly sitting in the big chair, and "The All Stars Poker Game" was on ESPN on television. We were entering a time where he could not distinguish the television from reality. I had to turn the TV off most of the time because he would believe that what he saw or heard on TV was happening to us. The news was especially dangerous, and sports … well, after watching a game, he would spend the whole night recruiting men for players on his team. He even designed sandwiches for Martha Stewart. I looked at a beautiful sandwich on which he had made a happy face and then carefully moved it into place to make room for the "chips on the side to even out the plate." I said, "Honey, I don't know whether to laugh or cry." I laughed with him as he ate his beautiful sandwich with chips on the side, and then I turned away and cried.

Where were we headed?

Sugar, our big white cat that came with me to our marriage, was now nearing nineteen years old. She was not a "lap cat," in fact, she was rather nasty. Don was never fond of her, and she rarely, if ever, approached him. But as he became incapacitated, I would come home to find her on his chest as he slept, or at his head, as though she was watching over him. At times, after a delusionary episode, he would say, "Sugar and I worked it out"! We began to call Sugar his "nanny cat."

Don began to have aphasia, which is the inability to correctly form words. We had a property for sale on a street called Yale. I asked him if he would like to go with me to show it one day, and he tried very hard to slip back into his old real estate broker self; he referred to the street as "Yalla." He could not tell he wasn't saying the words correctly. He was not able to fill the car up with gas. He could not drive to the most familiar places.

Don began to have trouble taking care of his physical needs. He said none of the many new razors we bought would work; the shower wouldn't turn on. He would forget where the bathroom was. He would go into the closet and try to put on my clothes. The appliances were all broken and wouldn't run. I taped a sign on his bathroom mirror that said "Shave, Shower, Brush" so he could remember what to do in the bathroom, but soon the words made no sense to him. He would become confused and unable to take care of himself appropriately.

We spent many hours in doctor's offices. While in one of them, Don had a moment when he became very strange. He looked ashen and vacant. The doctor said to me, "He has been through so much" that this was not surprising. When we reached the car, Don told me that while in the doctor's office, he saw a vision of an old truck stopped out in the country. The door was opened, and there was a blond-headed boy of about ten, in overalls, getting out of the truck. His voice broke and he began to sob as he said, "That boy was me." He had seen himself, and this vision had a most emotional effect on him. I had never seen my husband weep. He wept over that vision. He retold it many times, always with the same emotional effect. I wanted this vision to have purpose. I wanted it to have profound meaning. I wanted it to be healing. I couldn't, although I tried to, imagine what it was about this vision that affected him so.

I wanted to see it, too.

The Other Carols

November 8, 2006

Life doesn't get any less complicated. I am in midair, barely hanging on. I'm afraid and lonely. Every day—every night—is unpredictable and strange. Most of the time Don doesn't know me. He knows I'm his wife and that he loves me, but—damn—he doesn't know my name, and continually asks me how old I am and where I'm from! Today he asked me if I had any children. I said one, Rob, and he said he had a son named Rob, too. It breaks my heart. I can't imagine how it must feel to Don. He makes love to me and we are strangers. (from my journal)

We were on our way to the psychologist's office. The neurologist had required psychological testing before proceeding with his diagnosis. Don liked the psychologist and enjoyed talking to Dr. R about his thoughts and ideas. When we first started seeing Dr. R, Don had not been cooperative. He didn't want to talk, and he sure as heck wasn't going to be tested! I got him there, but he refused to do the tests, so Dr. R proceeded to evaluate him with verbal conversations. That went fairly well, over a period of weeks. There were times when Don just refused to get in the car at all, and so I went alone and sat in the psychologist's office, spilling my insides instead of Don. But on this trip across town, Don began to talk to me about "his wife," and he talked as though he didn't mean me. I said, "That was your first wife. Where is your present wife, Carol?" He looked right at me, and said, "I don't know. She just went away, and I don't know where she is." I felt like we had hit a semi-truck in the back at seventy miles an hour. What was I to say? What was I to think? I asked him who it was that was driving him, and he said, "A friend? A neighbor?" My husband didn't know me. How does one process that information?

In the doctor's office, we related this experience, and Don said a woman drove him there who was wearing a red jacket. There I sat next to him, in my red leather jacket. I thought my heart was going to break. It became more frequent then for him not to recognize me. Sometimes he would forget my name, and then sometimes he would talk about "the other Carol." It seemed to me that he could not differentiate between my roles. He would ask, "Are you the Carol that runs the office, or the one who takes care of me at home?"

Around Christmas, we took my granddaughter, Erin, to a movie, which he slept through. The next day, he was very agitated, and I thought going out to lunch would help him calm down. At the table in the diner, he seemed to slip into a different persona, and he asked me, "Will you get in trouble for having lunch with me?" He was using his business voice. He asked me how long I'd been with the organization and was I married, and he began telling me about a movie he had recently seen with Erin, his granddaughter (and I thought he had slept through it). He did not mention me being there at all, and I asked him if they went alone. He said, "No, someone who was with Erin went, too. It was someone connected to her." I was becoming a nonexistent person. I wanted to be at least as real as his invisible friends!

When we went to bed together, it was even worse. It seemed he would forget who he was laying with and ask me unthinkable questions, or call me by another name. This was overwhelming to me. I visualized myself melting away into the sheets and running off the bed to the floor and disappearing. The confusion about who I was happened so often that the experiences all ran together—and those times were impossible for me to not take personally. I was a stranger; the neighbor; a visitor; a nameless sexual partner. I was forgotten, and I was lonely for my husband.

When he could not remember my name, he not only knew I was hurt, but it hurt him, also. Researchers believe that our brain stores and processes memories of emotions differently from memories of fact. It is possible for the dementia to damage one without damaging the other as much. Once he was sad that he just could not call me by name, and as he held me he said, "I may not remember your name, but my heart knows it loves you." I wrote those words on my own heart and called on them repeatedly over the next months for comfort.

Our pillow talk in those days was often about God. Don seemed fearful that he had been a bad person and that the after-life was uncertain for him. He was confused about his relationships and often said he had been "a bad husband," for which he was sorry. He had forgotten about forgiveness. So we read the Bible and we talked of God's forgiveness, and we prayed together. He always brightened with new hope when we opened the Bible and read the words of salvation and prayed. One day during a particularly upsetting moment for him, Don suddenly turned to me with a huge smile, as though he remembered the answer, and said, "Let's read the Bible!" That act seemed to make him feel peaceful and comforted, even joyful.

Dr. R said several times that Don must have been a very powerful man and very much in control. He felt many of his actions were coming from the loss of control he was feeling. The three of us talked about this together. The day of the red-coat incident, when Don seemed so confused in the doctor's office, we talked of how strong I knew Don to be and how much I loved that in him. Don and I had a favorite story of the ancient city of Masada in Israel, an impenetrable fortress built on a mountaintop. The Jews who inhabited it hoped to be invulnerable to their enemies, but as the Romans drew closer, escape was impossible, and the Romans would be entering the city in the morning. The Jewish people made a pact that rather than be taken as slaves or face the brutality and torture of the Romans, they would die. When the enemy entered the city, they would find only dead bodies and would garner no spoils. The story of Masada was one Don and I had talked about for years, as it was a hallmark of love, courage, resolve, and strength—against insurmountable odds—even in the face of death, which I found in Don. Don listened as we talked in the office that day.

In the car on the way home from Dr. R's office, Don sat silently and then he turned to me and quietly said, "You were wrong about me in there. *I would have found a way to take you off the mountain.*"

Months later, as I stood on the ruins of the city of Masada, through Don's eyes I looked for a way of escape. I could see him intently searching and thinking and planning, as I'd seen him do in many seemingly hopeless situations before, absolutely sure that he would have found that way to get me off the mountain; so great was his resolve, power, courage, and love.

Carol Who Works at the Office

I was exhausted. I was frustrated and confused. It was easier for me to be angry, because when I stopped being angry, I cried relentlessly. I despised the management company, and I resented Don for ever starting it, and I couldn't explain how he had let it get so far out of control. I was angry that I was left to fix it and didn't know how. I wanted to blow it up with a great explosion that would send the records, or lack thereof, to Timbuktu! This monster had stolen all of my time, all my resources, my peace of mind, and my own business for the past year. And now Don had become distrustful of me and would not sign anything that required his signature … unless Carla said he should! I have to admit, this annoyed me, and I did not know where his distrust was coming from. He thought I was withholding the financial information about the company from him. I considered this part of his growing paranoia, but told him he could see anything he wanted. He asked for the check registers, so I brought them home to him, even though I knew that he could not comprehend what he looked at. Of course, the registers are an essential part of everyday business, and when I looked for them to take them back, he had hidden them and wouldn't tell me where they were. I found them locked in his vehicle, under the seat. Very soon, I learned that Don's paranoia was being fed a regular diet of suspicion by his children.

For a year, I had been working all day long at the management office and then coming home to do my oil and gas accounting, sometimes late into the night. My clients were trying to be patient, but I wasn't sure I could ever get them caught up. Oil and gas accounting is all about taxes, so as the end of the year approached, I was worried and simply did not know if I could have everyone's deadlines met. I was taking no money out of the management company, so the only income we had was my accounting income. If I spent all my time on the management company, I didn't get a paycheck, and I was getting scared.

Chuck, who came as such a blessing to the company, stood to have a ready-made business handed over to him if he would accept the deficit. He was good at the management business and liked it. It fit him. He was thirty-two that summer, which was six years younger than my son. I understand that Don must have felt threatened by this terrible situation; he was losing his business to someone else. I understand that none of his life made any sense anymore, and it may have seemed that Chuck and I were the ones denying him his business. Again Don began to imagine that I was being unfaithful, this time with Chuck. He told his children that we were having an affair. As in the past, nothing I could say swayed him, and frankly, I didn't have the time or energy to fight too much on this one. It seemed so absurd, not even a man with a psychosis would truly believe that one, I thought. When Don talked of it to Carla in my presence, even she assured him that it was not true. I was thankful for her support on that day, but that was short-lived.

I hired my niece to work in the management office, and she was invaluable during this transition. I had to pay a lot of debt off with my own money to get the company saleable. I was using every source I could to get myself out of the everyday running of the company so I could begin to work gainfully again. I had unfiled taxes due. My life seemed overwhelming. Every time I left Don alone, his calls would frighten me. I tried to have someone stay with him when I was gone all day, and it usually was Carla. Kate's husband, Larry, worked near our home, and he seemed to understand Don's condition better than anyone. He would stop in and see how Don was when his guard was down.

Dementia patients seem to have an uncanny ability to "fake" it. Old social skills and the ability to make customary social remarks are often retained longer than insight or judgment. Many of them are very intelligent—I have even heard nurses and doctors say that the more intelligent they are, the worse dementia seems to hit them. I imagine it is really that because of their intelligence, there is just more of a contrast to the before-and-after. At any rate, Don could take control of a visit and manipulate conversation and his actions so that the visitor would go away saying, "He's still old Don!" After he had lovingly hugged them good-bye, many times he would say, even about his own children, "Who the hell was that?"

But Larry came when Don was unprepared, and Don did not know him. Larry saw the dire straights we were in. He said he was keeping Don's condition and what I told him from Kate because she tended to overreact. I told him once that I was so glad he saw the real situation because I was afraid the way Don was able to fake it, if he got really sick, people might think I was poisoning him. We both laughed at the absurdity of that!

Don was manipulative in his psychosis. He would not want me to leave in the morning and would feign any situation to keep me at home. If that's what it took, he would even start an argument. By the time I finally left, I would be in tears and was worried sick about how Don would be at home alone. I would often call Larry as I left and ask him to come over and check on his father-in-law or have lunch with him. He always seemed happy to do so, and it made my day a little easier.

I set my goal to have my entire office moved home and functioning by the first of December 2006, so I could be home with Don. The day we moved the office, Don assumed he would help. Don had always been the worker; the muscle; the one who made things happen. He expected this of himself and pushed himself even as his strength and stamina diminished. We packed his truck with furniture and files and started loading the next truck before we noticed he was gone.

We found him at another office location with a large gash on his arm (which he seemed unaware of), struggling to unload the heavy furniture all by himself and completely disoriented. I took Don home while Rob and Chuck finished the move. I set my office up and had arranged with most of my clients to do their work in my home office. I would only have to be out of the house one day a week for work, and I knew I would need that time away from the situation for my own sake as well. I was prepared to employ whatever help I might need to care for Don if and when the time came, but at this point, I felt he would be well cared for with me at home.

We had a business to sell. Don and I had talked in the past about whether a business such as the management company had any value and where that value was. Chuck and I talked money and had a dollar figure in mind for the sale of the company. As time went by and I began to see the disastrous shape the business was in financially, I talked to James, Carla's attorney husband, about how to sell a company with such a deficit. I also sought counsel from a CPA I worked with in the oil and gas business. The conclusion was that if the buyer would accept the deficits, the only thing to sell was the meager office trappings. Even that was offset with contract advertising expenses that were yet unfulfilled. Don's company had no saleable value. If truth be known, I would have willingly *paid* just to get out of it.

Chuck was formally taking over the management business on January 1, 2007, and we had bank accounts to transfer, contracts to change over, a new office for the management company to set up and organize, not to mention landlords and tenants to assure the business was going on.

When I was a child, we used to play on what were called monkey bars. We would move across the track, one hand over the other, our feet never touching the ground. During this time, I felt like I was in the middle of the monkey bars … hanging by one hand as I swung to the next bar, hoping I wouldn't lose my grip as my feet dangled far off the ground. From day to day, I wasn't always sure I would make it to the next bar.

I had agreed to help in the transition of the business. Being a real estate agent, I had knowledge of tenant/landlord laws and accounting, and I had some exposure (through Don) to most of the clients. I knew some history and knew most of the people, as I had either been in the office to meet them or accompanied Don into the "wor" zone. Also, just being older and having Don's name gave me a certain authority that was needed to help Chuck settle into the new ownership. So I expected to be called on frequently, but I hoped and prayed that it would not be for very long. Chuck was finding his own bearings, and the time I had to spend there was waning. Still, every time the phone rang, I braced myself and was so tempted not to answer.

When I did have to be gone from home, about one day a week, Carla would come over and stay with Don. Sometimes, I would come home after a short grocery run or from a business errand to find both Kate and Carla there, both cars in the driveway, as though they had rushed over and didn't expect me back. They never explained why, and I didn't feel it necessary to ask, but I often wondered why they always seemed to show up during the few minutes I was gone. I thought Don must have panicked and called them, although I wondered why he didn't call me if he forgot where I was. Or maybe they had instructed him to call them if I left the house. But when the girls were there, I never worried about him or gave much thought to it. I was simply thankful that they were there for their father when he needed them. I knew they would talk of the farm, and old times, and people I had never met. I knew they would take care of him. Of course, the girls knew of his problems with the Carols and with home. I told them about everything that we were going through. All of that was entering into the research they were doing as we worked together on Don's behalf.

Home

Being in the real estate business, we had a little heads-up on house hunting. We were comfortable in my condo for thirteen years while we waited for just the right home for us. I wanted an old house with a lot of history and character, and Don wanted a house that required *no work*. Nothing we ever saw fit that bill. Several years earlier, I had sold a house in an area I had fallen in love with, and I took my mother to see the neighborhood. As we walked around that house, I told her that I wished we had bought that house for ourselves, and she said she wished we had bought it, too. Just a few months after that, in November 2001, my mother fell ill and died. My inheritance from her left me with enough money to buy the house of my choice. In 2002, the house right next door to the one I had showed my mother went on the market. I think I was the first real estate agent to see it, and we bought it. We were both thrilled and settled in for the rest of our lives.

 Our cottage-like home is located in a picturesque neighborhood, a remote little area with a beautiful lake in our back yard, and a creek along one side where wildlife of all kind lives. The creek is spanned by a nostalgic covered bridge. Huge, old oak, maple, weeping willow, and birch trees thrive on the lake. We had an abundance of forest creatures that bear their young every year and bring them to feed under our huge oak tree, where we made a special area for seed and food: our "feeding tree." We fed the ducks and geese, the songbirds and crows, the squirrels, the wild turkey, and even the raccoon and opossum. In the winter, we saw antlered deer in the yard against the snow, and in the fall we saw young fawns frolic in our yard. A stray peacock came one spring and stayed until midwinter, eating out of my hand and leaving me his precious feathers as a thank you gift. Our grandchildren caught fish and huge turtles in the lake and spent many hours in the paddleboat. If we were to grow old and possibly have to be confined to home, this was the place we both wanted to be.

But during the "other Carols" days, Don also began to be confused about "home." He would look inconsolably lost. He would say, just like a tired child who longs for his bed, "Let's go home." To look into his lost eyes made me despair, and I was dismayed at how to answer him. We *were* home. There was no place to go. Sometimes I would say, "Okay, honey. Get your coat on and we'll go," and I would drive around familiar places, look at neighborhoods lit up brightly with Christmas lights, or go out for ice cream; and when the garage door went up, he seemed to be satisfied that he was home. Until the next time.

Sometimes he begged. Sometimes he was desperately lost. Again, I tried to make sense of it. I thought maybe he wanted to go back to the farm home of his childhood. That house had burned down long ago, with only the dilapidated barn standing precariously beside the broken windmill. But I still wanted to know where it was he wanted to go. Did he want to go back to the house where he raised his children? To our old condo where we lived together for so long?

Sometimes he said this was not our house, but was a *replica* of our house, that we were renters and the landlord was going to be mad if I cleaned (or if I didn't clean). One Saturday, I was cleaning our bedroom and he became terribly upset that I was moving things, and he thought the landlord would be furious. He became so agitated that I thought he needed a change of scenery. We called Kate and Carla to come take him out for lunch. That seemed to break his train of thought, and we got past that one. Or so I thought.

It is the job of the sane to calm the madness, is it not? I was toughening up so that I did not fall apart when Don's actions or words cut me to the bone. I kept telling myself that it was "not about me" and that this was his illness. "Do not take it personally" became my mantra. What must it feel like to want to go home; what was behind the pleading eyes, the hell he must be feeling to be so lost? Perhaps it was that he had lost himself; that he didn't recognize who he was anymore. Perhaps he meant "I want to go back to the condition of life, the quality of life when everything seemed to have a purpose and I was useful; someplace familiar where I will feel like myself again." Of all the changes that were going on in our lives, I think this was the hardest for me, because there was no answer to this question. No way to comfort him; no place to take him and make it all better. I, too, wanted to go home ... and home for me was where he was, and he wasn't *there* anymore.

I kept nothing from Don's children, telling them of his confusion with the Carols and with home, and his increasingly dark hallucinations. Sometimes they would say, "Oh, he is such a tease!" and I wondered what they thought I was telling them. Kate would always come up with a slough-off answer to what I told her. Even when Don would exhibit his actions in her presence, she would find a way to dismiss it. Kate and Carla accompanied us to doctor's appointments when they could, so they were made fully aware of the reality of the seriousness of his condition.

By the fall of 2006, we had all seen drastic changes in Don. In September, he was becoming frightened to go out—maybe frightened that he would not act appropriately. For some time, he had been uncomfortable around all but a few people. By October, his confusion made him unable to drive. He couldn't find his way home, and he couldn't seem to remember how to maneuver the car. In November, the hallucinations increased. By Christmas, he was paranoid and had become distrustful of me. He was losing all touch with reality, and by then, we were seeing psychologists and psychiatrists regularly. Don's two daughters, Kate and Carla, and I had been working together to try to find something that made sense. But we still had few answers, and Don got worse every day. On Christmas Day, I was alone with Carla for a moment and told her of some of Don's recent behaviors. She hugged me as I wept. I felt comforted that I could tell her such intimacies. She asked if we had the resources to put Don in a nursing home, or could we sell some assets if we needed to. The words *nursing home* sobered me up quickly! I did not want to hear those words and was not ready to even consider that an alternative. I told Carla I had given this serious thought and I was going to keep Don at home—others we knew of had done this, and it didn't seem impossible for me to achieve. I told her unless he became violent, which was so against his character that I wasn't worried about that ever happening, I was going to take care of him at home. We had just concluded the move of my office to our home so I could be with Don all the time.

I also confided to her that we were about to close on the sale of farmland in Oklahoma that Don had inherited but that he could no longer take care of, and that the sale would provide any money needed should he need care.

That Christmas night, Don and I lay in our bed holding each other and thanking God for the peace and love of our family and that we were blessed to be one of the few blended families that loved each other.

As Don lay sleeping, I lay awake thinking over the day as I always do before falling asleep. And I remembered something puzzling: "What was it Carla had said to me today that had stunned me for a moment?" Oh yes, when I was in her embrace after confiding in her my greatest disappointments, she had asked me, "Do you want a divorce?"

> *December 4, 2006*
>
> *I don't know if Don's condition worsens, but it constantly changes. He's losing himself so quickly, and the hope of recovery has left me. I don't know if I'm more afraid of his dying, or of his living like this. For now—if things could stay the same—it is not so bad. Although he is not well and he is confused, he is happy and loving and content most of the time. But the nature of this illness is to not remain so. Everyone is sad to see him no longer what he was, and he is saddest of*

all. I wish I could control my sadness and tears better, for his sake. It just overwhelms me and I find it hard to stop crying. He will say to me, "I won't be here" for this or that. It's not that I will be alone ... it's that I won't be with him. (from my journal)

Laughter and Despair
2007

Our house was always full of laughter. Don was fun to be with. We laughed a lot together. He was witty and would say the most surprising things. He made me laugh at myself. He seemed to see the world through different eyes than me. We would challenge each other with bets and dares, and the prize was always our laughter. We *enjoyed* each other, and we enjoyed being together. We were like children playing together. We teased each other and laughed at our private jokes, of which there were many. Everything was fair game to us. We were out one evening with nothing in particular in mind when Don spotted an ice cream shop. He made a quick turn into the drive-through, which wound around the back of the building. As we rounded the curve, there was an ice cream cone the size of a man to our left. I told Don, "That's where you order," and he stopped and gave his lengthy order to the ice cream cone. I let him go through the whole spiel before saying, "Don, you are talking to an ice cream cone. The order window is there," and pointed to the lady hanging out the window trying to hear his order. We both laughed like the good friends we were at something that was really funny.

The sadness of losing someone you love, inch by inch, can be devastating. I could not afford to despair and still be there for Don. When he did something funny, I could not act as though he was fragile and would be offended if I laughed. Dementia does not suddenly end a person's capacity to experience love or joy, or laughter. Happiness may seem out of place in the face of trouble, but laughter is a gift to help us keep our sanity. I wanted to enjoy every part of him that I could and to help him laugh at himself.

I always thought Don's children lacked a sense of humor, but never so much as after he got sick. In fact, they seemed to think that humor at that stage was blasphemous and chided me if I laughed at anything that happened or that Don did. Mostly, I think they had a misconception of who their father was. They certainly did not understand the relationship that Don and I enjoyed.

Our lives went on that fall and winter, with everyday things happening, and I coveted the moments when one of us would do something that we could laugh at. And there were many opportunities for that. I would laugh and, if need be, explain to Don what had happened that was funny. A smile would begin around his eyes, and then he would feel clever and "normal" again. He seemed to know that his "girlfriend" still found him fun to be with.

My sister and her husband were visiting one evening in February. Don seemed to be slipping into a new phase, which had become characteristic of his illness. I wasn't sure yet what this phase would bring, but on this particular evening, he seemed agitated and confused. For the most part, he sat quietly as we chatted; a televised ballgame droned on in the background. I thought he must be watching the ballgame, or at least listening to it. All of a sudden, he started to speak, but his words didn't make sense. As he continued to ramble on, my mind began to wonder. Don's voice became ever more passionate as he spoke, but still his words made no sense. At this point, I was beginning to feel a little uncomfortable, especially for our company. Then without warning, Don stopped and said, very articulately, "… and we pray these things in Jesus' name!"

He had our full attention at that point, and I could not keep back my laughter! My sister and her husband did well to sit quietly, but I lost it. Don looked at me and began to laugh, too. I doubt he knew what was so funny, but it was just good to see him laugh and feel funny again. Then we all began to laugh together. As for

Don, I sensed he needed to feel connected, that he was still fun to be with, and that he was a normal person enjoying a fun evening with friends.

Sometimes, he said and did hilarious things. Sometimes, it was from pure frustration at people or situations. If he ever had any inhibitions, he lost them. He spoke his mind, and it made me laugh. The things he said were witty and very clever. His children chided me for laughing at what he said or did. They even called it "emotional abuse." We laugh at the things our children do and say, and we tell other family members, and sometimes strangers, of their cleverness. We repeat the funny stories and find it endearing. To cease laughter at this period of our lives would seem a cruel punishment. We are told that *laughter is the best medicine,* and for me there is no better road to health than to laugh away some of the despair.

For us, in the days to come there would be precious little to raise even a flicker of a smile.

The Diagnosis

The obvious diagnosis was Alzheimer's. Although there was certainly dementia, there were too many things that didn't fit Alzheimer's. Besides, *Alzheimer's* was a word that brought terror to me, and I was not going to give in to it. Doctors would say that word, and I felt it was a word of dismissal, synonymous with "in the trash basket." We continued to do research and I read of a disease called "Lewy body dementia" (LBD). As much as it shocked and terrified me, from living with his daily symptoms, I knew immediately that this was what Don was suffering from.

Whereas Alzheimer's, simply put, is degeneration or disconnection of brain cells, for which the major symptom is memory loss, Don was experiencing the classic symptoms of schizophrenia: hallucinations, delusions, and separation from reality (psychosis). He was also showing increased signs of Parkinson's disease: the dragging gait, slumping posture, facial "mask," and extremity pain. His memory did not seem to be affected; it was his disassociation with reality and the fluctuating cognition. As with the Carols, it was not that he didn't *remember* me, but that he didn't *recognize* me and our relationship.

After I read about Lewy body, I covered my face in my hands and wept. It was like seeing a terrible, fatal accident; you cannot take your eyes from it, yet simultaneously you cannot bear to watch. Lewy body proteins (named after the scientist Friederich H.

Lewy) are abnormal protein deposits that disrupt the brain's normal functioning. These proteins are deposited in an area of the brain stem, causing Parkinson's. In Lewy body dementia, these abnormal proteins are diffuse throughout other areas of the brain, including the cerebral cortex. The result is a disruption of perception, thinking, and behavior. LBD is a combination of dementia and Parkinson's. Like Alzheimer's, there are no physical tests to diagnose it, but according to experts, it can be diagnosed if two of the following three symptoms are present: 1) fluctuation of cognition and alertness, 2) recurrent visual hallucinations, and 3) Parkinsonian symptoms. After that, there are twenty-two more symptoms; Don had every single one.

Treatment of LBD is difficult once it is diagnosed. First of all, it is a relatively newly recognized disease (1996), and many doctors do not know about it. When I mentioned it to several of Don's doctors, they were not aware of it and had to look it up. Medical management is complex because of increased sensitivity to many drugs. Many of the medications regularly given to Alzheimer's and Parkinson's patients can adversely affect people with LBD. Many neuroleptic drugs, sedatives, and medications useful for Parkinsonian symptoms may increase confusion, delusions, and hallucination. We found out the hard way that Don had adverse reactions to many sedatives, such as Lortab and even Benedryl. And drugs such as Ativan would cause him to enter a violent psychosis. If a doctor or caretaker does not understand these things, or accept the diagnosis, the result can be terrible.

I had no idea how to care for Don. We were in a horrifying situation, for which there was no map. Even for the doctors, it is trial-and-error. I knew I loved him and I would do the best I could for him; that's about all I knew. In this wilderness, I was following every direction in which the doctors pointed us. In the midst of this confusion, where it seemed as if the blind were leading the blind, I studied dementia, specifically LBD, and consulted with every physician I could. Don was taking several medications prescribed by the cardiologist for his heart, cholesterol, and blood pressure. He was taking drugs for nausea prescribed by his gastroenterologist.

He was taking antidepressants and antianxiety drugs prescribed by the gerontologist, and sedatives, cognitive drugs, and Parkinson's drugs prescribed by the psychiatrist; he was also taking B-12 shots, vitamins, and aspirin. And he had not yet been diagnosed with LBD. The girls and I were sure there were problems with the dosage or correct drugs, but we didn't know what to do about it. The doctors were watching him closely and trying out different drugs at every turn, constantly adjusting his dosage to see if anything would help him.

Although I was sure Don had LBD in the fall of 2006, he was not diagnosed until April of 2007. Even then, his neurologist tiptoed around it until I asked, "You are trying to tell me he has Lewy body dementia, aren't you?" He looked at me with complete surprise that I would know that, and finally said the words.

LBD is a very fast-paced disease, and people who have it do not live but three to seven years from onset, as a rule. With Alzheimer's, the prognosis can be up to twenty-two years. In just a few months, Don had declined so rapidly that in April, the doctors said he was in the early last-stages of the disease.

I had seen this before. Back then (not so very long before Don became sick), it didn't have a name. The doctors said it must be Parkinson's, but there were so many other complications. Don and I had gone to visit Bobby, Don's older brother, in the hospital several times. The time we spent there was unbearable for me. Bobby was mean and demanding, but I tried to overlook it because he was obviously in pain. He would cry out for something to ease the aching in his legs. He would cry out to Don over and over, "Help me, Donnie, help me."

Bobby held his body in a certain way, just as Don was holding his body now. Bobby's face had taken on a stony look—with no expression, just as Don's face had settled into a permanent lack of expression. Bobby had lost control of his bodily functions. He was in the hospital but the doctors were at a loss to know what to do for him. He was moved to a nursing home, and after a short time, he died.

The Sound of a Dropping Shoe

Just after noon, on Friday, February 9, 2007, I returned home after working at the management office. Carla had been with Don most of the day. I found them sitting quietly and solemnly together on the couch. Carla was very sober, and I wondered what secrets they must have been sharing that were so gloomy. I didn't even try to find out or guess what the morning had been like. Don had called me several times throughout the morning, asking me when I would be home, and he seemed to be very happy that I was back, as Carla abruptly got up and left. The next day, Don was agitated and bored, and he said he would like to go out for a late lunch. He chose one of our long-favorite restaurants. After we had ordered, Don felt he couldn't sit there any longer. His level of anxiety had skyrocketed instantly. He walked around the restaurant awhile and was able to eat a little of his food before we left. He slept most of the remainder of the day.

In Kansas, the dark winter skies often look like actual snowdrifts, but no snow falls. Sunday, February 11, was just such a day. Don was pacing, and there was nothing that interested him. When he was like this, he would follow me around, staring at me, hovering as if he were going to crawl onto my back. I had gotten somewhat used to it. I had so much work to do that I was constantly looking for every moment I could go to my desk. So when Don was quiet, I made my way down to my office. On this dark afternoon, he followed me there and sat in the overstuffed chair in front of my desk, where he always sat. Classical music was playing, and to the constant whirr of the calculator, Don fell asleep.

When he awoke, it was late afternoon, but with the grey and somber skies, it could have been midnight. Don awoke disoriented, confused, and lost. He wanted to "go home." Although it does no good, the first reaction is to try to rationalize: "We *are* home, Don. This is your home. Where do you want to go?" As he relentlessly begged to go home, his tone became desperate, and I began to cry for lack of any answer. It hurts to know that this person you love doesn't recognize the home you have made together and does not recognize you as the heart of that home. I had reached the point of being distraught myself. And when it goes on and the passion and anxiety heightens, there is no more conversation to have. The expression on his face showed the agony of being completely lost. I was his only hope of getting home, and I had nothing to offer. As though he felt abandoned with no shelter at all, the last thing he said to me was, "I will pay for a place to stay tonight." His desperation was tangible, but I had no answer. Fleetingly, I thought of packing a bag and going to a motel, but I knew a strange place would have only further confused him. And then he turned from me and went up the stairs. A million times since, I have thought, "What could I have done differently?"—with no reasonable answer.

I felt about as desperate as he and needed a minute to collect myself. I thought, *I will put my work away and take him out to a drive-through; any change of pace.* He had been upstairs about ten minutes when I walked up. He was standing at the top of the stairs with his coat on. I said, "Are you cold?" and he answered no. I said, teasingly, "Are you going someplace?" and he said yes. Just then his cell phone rang. After a short few seconds, with no conversation on his end, he hung up. I was thinking this was all very strange, when at that moment Larry, Kate's husband, came through the front door. I started to speak to Larry, but his voice was strained and anxious, and he yelled, "Come on, Don, right now! Come on, let's go!" Don turned and said he was going to get a glass of tea that he had just made to take with him, but Larry insisted, "No! Leave it." Then Don came to me, embraced me, and started to kiss me, but Larry grabbed him away from my arms ... and they were gone. Gone! Larry was driving a little red car, and as I saw it speed away, the leaden sky turned bright red. Even now, when I think of that dreadful afternoon, everything in my head is as red as blood.

I stood alone in my house, with the front door standing open. I felt like a cartoon character, left spinning in the wake of a whirlwind that came out of nowhere. *What the hell?* I thought. *What has just happened?* I was sick to my stomach. I tried to figure out what had taken place and why. Maybe Don had called one of the kids to come take him to dinner—but the way this happened didn't make any sense. Surely they would be back in a while.

I tried not to panic. I tried the word *maybe* with every conceivable idea. I didn't want to read too much into what had just happened. Don was not upset when he left; he had embraced me and kissed me; his glass of tea sat untouched on the counter. There was no reason to think this was any more than a badly carried-out effort to take Dad out for a while. I had no choice but to wait in the silence of our home, trying to control an indefinable, sinister feeling that threatened to overcome me.

Late in the evening, Carla called and said Don wanted to spend the night at Kate's. She said he was upset and didn't want to come home. He hadn't seemed upset when he left with Larry, but I understood that with the delusions he was having lately, there was no telling what he was experiencing. Also, like a child, he was happiest where he got the most attention. With Carla, James, Kate, Larry, and their children, he would be getting plenty of attention. Carla came by to pick up an overnight bag. When she did, she seemed confused herself, but just said her father didn't want to come home yet; they didn't know why. She added that he did not want to talk to me either. She just said, "We will take care of him." She never asked me if something had happened, and I had nothing to explain. This was all very frightening and disarming. I could think of no reason on earth why he should feel this way, unless he was having a psychosis, and surely the kids would recognize that. I thought it would pass. Carla said they would call me tomorrow. I closed the door behind Carla and stood against it, frozen with apprehension for the long night that was ahead. I suddenly realized I was afraid of these people.

I could not work the next day, Monday. I waited all morning, but no one called. I gave them until midafternoon, and then I called our son-in-law Larry; Larry, who *knew* what was going on. He would be honest with me. He would understand. He would explain why he had taken Don. But I was wrong. Larry was evasive and would not answer any question I asked him. He said he just didn't know anything and it would be better if I didn't call again; that I should just leave Don alone. *Leave my husband alone?* I was too distraught to insist and too afraid of them to push it further. It would work out. Don would get over whatever it was, and he would come home. By evening, I was about to go mad. My world had changed in an instant … with no explanation. Don had left with nothing. That meant he was coming back! Yes. I would hear from him soon. I did not say anything to anyone. But I was dying inside, and the not-knowing was the worst of it.

I could not sleep Monday night. I sat up for hours, weighing every conversation, every action for the past week, trying to think what I could have done, or what Don could have done that would have caused such action on the part of his children. At two in the morning, I sat down to e-mail the girls and beg them to talk to me.

> *E-mail dated February 13, 2007, 3:24 am*
>
> *Larry, Kate, Carla: By now, we all know that we are in for a very difficult time ahead with Don. Things may be progressing faster than any of us thought, or maybe it just crept upon us and we didn't see how severe it was getting—although I live with him, pretty much 24 hours a day, and I have been experiencing the delusions and misconceptions he has for some time. For the past 36 hours I have been stunned, and scared, and completely alone with what happened on Sunday.*

Because I did not know what precipitated Larry coming to get Don, I assumed Don got upset and asked to go out for a while, as he has done at times. When he didn't come back, and then didn't WANT to come back, I was just baffled and waited to hear something that would make some sense of this.

As the hours wore on and no one communicated what was really going on, it got scarier for me. I called Larry and felt he was very careful about what he said to me. I called Carla later, and have been trying to figure what this was all about.

At this point, I do not know what Don told you when he called on Sunday. I did not know he even called anyone. When Larry came, he made no explanation and whisked Don away without allowing any conversation at all, and I was standing in the middle of the room not knowing what just happened.

Carla told me she is very protective of her dad, and acted out of that, and I respect that. But as I've sat for hours and thought over this, I wonder what you thought he needed protection from. And when I thought about the manner in which Larry took Don, I came to the conclusion that Don must have told you something happened that frightened you. I need you to tell me what that was ... because nothing did happen Sunday to cause this reaction.

Don is not a prisoner here. We have always had an open door policy with all of you kids, and I believe I have encouraged you all to be with Don as much as you wanted, or to do anything that you wanted with him—without reservation. I have been so happy that you have all loved Don and been close to him and you have helped us out so much by being willing to come get him or stay with him at a moment's notice. And I want to encourage that, because as time goes by, we will all need to be actively working to hold us all together and do what's best for Don.

But what will harm him the most is if we get a rift between us and lose trust in each other to work for his good. In the clarity of the night hours, it seems to me that you thought Don was being mistreated by me and was in some danger. Apparently he conveyed that idea to you. I hope that you will realize that he has a difficult time with reality and is often confused with what is happening or what has happened. We all know that for some time he has the problem of the "Carols" and with where home is. This is not likely to get any better, so we are going to have to come up with a way to cope with it. If it comes to the point that he doesn't want to live here with me, we will have to deal with that reality. In the meantime, I must feel that you do not perceive me as "the enemy." I think our love for each other has been evidenced over the years, and for me, that hasn't changed. I realize that—in a dispute—you would take his side, as you should, but you must at least consider that what he might tell you may not be reality. A lot of hurt may have been avoided if someone had called me and asked what was going on. I would not have tried to keep Don from going anywhere with any of you for any length of time, but I felt sucker-punched with what happened. I ask you to give me the benefit of the doubt and to communicate with me. Maybe if we could have talked about whatever he was feeling together, he could have been more clear about what was bothering him. I hope being away from home/me for a while is a positive experience for Don, but for me it has been devastating.

I still do not know what happened this week. And unless you want to talk about it, I am willing to let it go. But I need your trust that, although I will make mistakes with him, I will not harm him. I ask that

> *you communicate with me before you react. I will not stand in your way to be with him, or take him, but you must consider me in that decision. The hours that I have spent worrying, stewing, crying, and mourning are difficult to deal with, and I don't think I can go through this again. We will have to work closely together to find what is best for Don now. We have to trust each other and communicate with each other. What we don't need is anything that would come between me and you kids as we try to do this. I didn't think I could get past the emotion to say what I wanted to, thus the e-mail. I hope you will understand that I am trying to bring us together, not tear us apart. I love you all. Carol*

I checked my e-mail early and had a response from Carla. She said she had not slept through the night either and wanted to talk to me. I called her before 8:00 am. The conversation boiled down to this: the kids did not want to discuss anything with me; their intention was to put Don in a nursing home. I was not ready to hear that. The insistence upset me and in tears, I said I couldn't go on with this conversation. An e-mail later from Kate:

> *February 13, 2007*
>
> *Carol, while I totally understand your feelings I have to honor what my father wants at this point. My greatest concern for Dad is that HE makes the decision regarding what he wants; not what you and/or his children might or might not want. I think he is still capable of making those decisions; he just needs time.*
>
> *I want you to know that I understand your feelings and anxiety. Please take care of yourself and give this some time. I know Dad wants to talk to you at some point; however, I don't think he is quite ready. Please be patient with him. Again, take care of yourself. Kate*

I pled with her again:

> *February 13, 2007*
>
> *Kate, I am at a complete loss about what is going on. I don't know what you are talking about. No one has told me what Don's feelings are, or what the problem is. Please understand that I need some information. Apparently he is talking to you, but I am completely in the dark. Please tell me what is going on.*

I received no answer and no more civility from Don's children. It was as though they had decided, from that moment on, I did not exist.

Early on that Tuesday morning, the realization finally hit me then that I needed help. This was not an overnighter! I called my son, Rob, and told him what had happened. Not knowing what motive these people had or how far they would go, I felt completely vulnerable. They had stolen my husband; what else might they steal? Our first thought was that we should protect the money in my personal banking account from them. Don and I had always kept our money separate, even in separate banks, but our accounts were held in joint tenancy, as is the case in most marriages. We were at the bank when the doors opened, where I intended to move a good portion of my money into a personal account that I also kept.

But I was already too late.

The bank notified me that Carla had already taken Don into the banks and taken money out of all of our joint accounts, leaving two of the accounts overdrawn. I was stunned. I was worried about the business accounts. But I never dreamed to what extent they would take this. I have a rental property, my condo that I bought before Don and I were married. It is still in my maiden name. The rental banking account, however, was also held in joint tenancy. I remembered that and went directly to that bank. It too had been cleaned out. "I'm going to be sick," I said, and they took me to a back room as I began to collapse.

The weekend was approaching. My house was hauntingly lonely, and I was constantly afraid. I decided that I could not spend the time alone. I packed my little bag and went to spend the weekend with Rob and my grandchildren. It was February 17, and Don had been gone almost a week. His kids would not talk to me, and they said Don did not want to talk to me. The "WHY" of all this was driving me mad. I was sick. I was praying constantly that this nightmare would stop and life would make some sense again. I thought that if Don had confusion with who Carol was, and with home, maybe he would be better and happier with his children. If he did not know me as his wife, and yet was in bed every night with a "stranger," it would be better that he not be with me. I could accept that. I rationalized any way that made any sense. I tried to understand why he would be so upset with me that this could happen.

Kate finally e-mailed me that Don was not coming back. She asked me to pack Don's clothing and medicines, which I did. As I left for Rob's, I placed it on the porch for her to pick up. I took this opportunity to communicate and enclosed the following letter, still hoping to appeal to them:

> February 16, 2007
>
> For your information, the bank account from which you took money is our household account out of which I pay all living expenses, including groceries, Don's medications, mortgage, taxes, insurance, clothing, utilities, etc. You found that account as a joint account because Don and I are married, and we have always honored and trusted each other, but it is my personal account, made up of my income. By taking all of that account, you overdrew the account and all of my household checks have bounced. Although it is a joint account, Don has never accessed that account, does not carry those checks, nor manage that account. You have stolen MY money.
>
> The other account is also a joint account, simply because we are married, but it is Don's personal account. I had never accessed that account, written checks on it, nor managed it until the last six months when he

became unable to pay his bills. His Social Security, rent income and any other income he receives goes into that account. The only thing paid out of that account, ever, is his loan payments, farm expenses, etc. and HOA dues and any other expenses for his town home. By taking the money from that account, you have caused an overdraft for his monthly loan payment and HOA dues, and made it impossible for me to keep him solvent. In that account was also the rental security deposit for his town home.

I wonder how you expect me to continue meeting his obligations without access to his money. What you have done is a breach of our marriage covenant.

The mess you have made for me to clean up, and the humiliation to Don that will result as I have to resolve this with the banks and loan institutions, will be irreparable. Since I have known Don, there have been three things that are important to him: his family, me, and his financial integrity. You have robbed him of two of those. While saying you are "protecting" your father, you have exposed him to his worst fear, financial embarrassment, and you have made exposure of his inadequacies public.

On my way to Rob's Saturday morning, I felt physically sick. I thought I should stop by my clinic—if I could get in. In a silent prayer, I said, *If I can get right in, I will stop.* I was so distraught and in despair that I didn't think I could hold myself together long in the waiting room. I drove by and no one was there yet, and it was time for it to open. I was first in line so I knew the wait would not be long. My personal doctor, a lovely young woman, Rebecca, never works the ER, so I did not think I would be seen by anyone who knew me. I thought I could certainly be mistaken for a basket case by a stranger who didn't know of my situation. As I was led to an examining room, I was face-to-face with my doctor, Rebecca, as she waited for the first patient. She said it was one of the few times she had ever been called to work the ER. Behind the closed door, I began to sob and told her what had happened. She drew close to me, took my hands in hers, and began to pray. I was so distraught that I didn't hear her words until she prayed, "*Convict these children and make them see that their actions do not honor their father.*" That was a prayer I could not pray for myself, and those words became "Rebecca's prayer" to me. I recited her words in prayer over and over throughout the next months. I did not know a doctor could take the liberty to pray with a patient, but I was so blessed by her that day, and it was a sign to me that God knew what was happening in my life, that He cared, and that He was with me in the midst of this. I left the clinic with an antibiotic for tonsillitis and a new awareness that God was with me.

My son, Rob, was my hero. Although I tried not to think about what he was feeling inside, I knew if he chose to act, nothing could hold him down. He is not a pacifist. As far as he was concerned, his mother had been violated: raped, beaten, and left to die! But for my sake, he simply loved me and protected me. He was always there when I needed him, and he and his children provided me with comfort and embraced me completely. I was not the only one being violated. Don's children had also taken Rob's "Dad" from him, and Rob's children, Erin and Dalton, had lost their "Papa." In my mind, as I grow old there will forever be the picture of my son Rob as he opened the door to Erin's room, where we two had just snuggled into bed. I will never forget the security I felt as he said, "I just came in to say good night to my two best girls." As he turned out the light and pulled the door to, for the first time in many days I went to sleep with a smile on my face.

The next week, Don began calling me. Each time, he sounded ill and spoke in a monotone. He said he loved me and wanted to come home. He asked if we could "work it out." First we made a date to have dinner, which I thought was a reasonable start, but Carla said he could not go out with me. We made plans to see the psychologist together, but Carla wouldn't allow that either. We were being treated like children who required permission to see each other. Every time we even tried to talk, Kate or Carla would intervene and shut it down until he no longer called. They would not let me see him. I tried to go on with my life, which is the most difficult thing to do when your life is in the toilet. I went to the grocery store. I walked the familiar aisles and reached for the familiar things … fruit, sandwich meat, bread, the things that Don liked. I put them back. I didn't know how to buy groceries for me. I stood in the frozen food aisle and wept. I stood looking at the canned foods and wept. People passed me as I stood weeping, and I didn't care. I felt totally lost in a place so familiar. As I left the store, I looked in my basket, and I had three frozen dinners, one container of cottage cheese, and six small cans of tomato juice.

I don't like tomato juice.

As I left the store that day in tears, panic rose until I could taste its bitterness in my mouth. I called Carla as I drove, hardly able to see, and begged to see my husband, but she said without emotion that I could neither talk to him nor see him. And she hung up on me.

Sugar, Don's nanny cat, quit eating. In a few weeks, I would bury her under the snow in the cold flower bed beside our house.

The Law

Don and I were married in a church by a minister, in a legal ceremony. We became husband and wife on August 18, 1990. We established a home. We established a family. We were married in the truest sense of the word. The minister said, "No judge or minister can marry you. You marry one another." Those words have stayed with me through the years because they were true for us—Don and I truly married one another. We had made a covenant with God and with each other. We believed the laws required everyone else to recognize and honor our legal marriage. Traditional marriage vows conclude with "What God hath joined together, let no man tear asunder." We all believe the laws of our land uphold the marriage vows. The spouse is given the place next to her mate that supersedes the children. It was not possible that these adult children could kidnap my husband and I had no rights. The doctors said, "As Don's wife, you ultimately have the right to decide what is best." The attorney said, "In the courts the wife is given precedence over the children in such cases." We all remember the Terri Schiavo story, in which the husband was given precedence all the way through to the Supreme Court, even over her parents. So, I felt confident driving to my attorney's office that this would right itself.

However, I was not given much hope when I saw my attorney on that first day. As soon as the girls took Don, Carla had acquired a power of attorney (POA) from Don, and Kate had acquired a "medical power of attorney," and these both took precedence over any rights I might have as Don's wife. How could this be allowed to happen? My attorney explained to me that this was possible because the fact that Don was incapacitated had not yet been determined in a court of law; therefore, any legal documents with his signature would be honored. He said that I could start legal action against them, but that would take time, and God knows, this would surely end soon … these people are my family, after all! It was to no one's advantage to have this kind of division when Don needed us all. His advice was to try to find a way to settle this without taking it to court. For now, there was no intervention that could take place lawfully. Although the courts usually frown on any interference with a marriage relationship, it still has to reach the courts before that judgment can be made. My husband had been kidnapped, and I had no legal recourse.

Was this not America, where our whole society is based on marriage and family? If common decency fails, which it had, are there not laws that protect the marriage contract? Is it possible that someone outside a marriage can lawfully bring a marriage to an end against the wills of both spouses?

The small Oklahoma farm sale that I had told Carla about was scheduled to close the week of February 12. I called the Oklahoma Title Company to see when the check would be issued. From the bank, I had secured a lien release on the property, which was held as collateral, and part of the proceeds of the sale were designated to satisfy one of Don's bank debts. The check was to be sent registered mail to our home in both of our names. Initially, Don had inherited a substantial amount of acreage from his parents. He had sold the majority of it years ago to help pay his cattle debt. There was only a small portion of acreage left in his possession. To my knowledge, Don's children had no idea how much land we were selling, but they believed it was significantly greater than it was. I had been working for months on this sale, had made several trips to Oklahoma, and had talked many times to the title company office. This time when I called, their tone seemed different. I was told that they had received a power of attorney from Carla, and the check would be made out to Don alone, and it would go to Carla. Once again, I was stunned! That was $50,000 more gone, and the debt was still due. Again, although what they had done was not in line with the law, there was nothing I could do about it. All of our money was in someone else's account, and all of Don's debts were in mine. I felt like the lion that had chased the prey all day, caught my lunch, and then the jackals had stolen it from me.

I believe Carla's husband, James, was at the core of this action. He and Carla had never had children, had divorced once, and after several years remarried. He was a malpractice attorney of small stature but with a huge ego. In my opinion, for him, the law was all about winning and had nothing to do with what was right. Generally, the hope of the malpractice lawyer is to terrorize people with lawsuits to get a settlement instead of having to prove their case. He did not care that this was Don, or Carol, or Carla's family; it was a game that was to be won because he knew how. From beginning to end of this ordeal, James made sure that his name was not found on anything, but his "signature" was nevertheless on each and every legal move that was made.

Kate had said, in her last e-mail, "Take care of yourself." I had no idea at the time what she had meant by that, but it was becoming painfully clear. I was frightened and did not know to what lengths they would go to take other possessions. With James intimately involved, I expected they would go as far as he could find loopholes. I had worked and saved and had assets and money of my own, in my own name. I received notification from the attorneys demanding our tax information, my own personal financial information, an appraisal of our home, and the value of even our furniture! Their intent was obviously clear. I was desperate to find a way to protect my personal assets from Don's children. I decided the best way was to draw up a trust and put my personal assets in the trust. I did that, thinking that was a wise and prudent thing to do. I put my rental property and our home, which is also in my name only, in the trust. No jointly owned property was transferred to the trust. Within my trust was provision for my husband, Don, to be cared for with the corpus of the trust until his death. I was not attempting to keep anything from Don, only from his children.

Don's two primary doctors, his psychologist and gerontologist, were in the same office. I called to see if they could see me. They both were very interested in what was going on; they had recently seen Don and knew that something had happened, but said they didn't know what the situation was. So I made an appointment to see them both together. I assumed the girls had told the doctors their side of this event, which I needed to know. I was desperate to understand what had happened and what Don was feeling, and to get some instruction on how to proceed. I needed to know what was best for Don. I arrived Friday morning, February 16, and they both seemed to be acting differently than usual. I told them what I knew, and they told me nothing. Every time I asked about Don, they brought the subject back to me, as though I were their patient. Finally, dense as I was, they had to spell it out to me. The girls had *removed* me from Don's records and forbidden me to be given any information regarding him, his condition, or his treatment. Another door was slammed in my face. For a moment, I couldn't grasp what they were saying. I said, "But I *am* his wife. I *am* already on the papers." But Don's daughters had taken away all my rights, even to know if these doctors were still treating Don or not. The psychologist said, "How are you dealing with the anger, Carol?" I was so confused I didn't even know what I was supposed to be angry about. I felt totally betrayed. I felt exploited. And as I brushed past him on my way out the door, I said, "By cussing like a sailor—and I am physically sick. I am not your patient. I am here because I thought you could help me understand what is happening to Don, not to satisfy your curiosity. I've got real problems to solve and I don't have time for this nonsense!"

My next stop was to the banks, where I had to figure out what to do about thousands of dollars of overdrafts I could not cover.

The next week, I was grief stricken and distraught. I cried alone every night. I waited for the phone to ring, but it did not. I kept busy during the day working, but in the evenings, my moods were unpredictable. As our friends and family began to learn of what had happened, they were stunned and confused, and they rallied around me. It touched me deeply. Friends came by and brought me dinner, knowing I was not eating. They took me out, although that was tenuous, because I could rarely swallow my food as I choked on tears. Before, I never went out without Don, and now I found myself staring at a menu, thinking we always shared a meal, so how do I order? My family would call or come over and cry with me. Everyone wanted to *do* something but there was nothing to do. Some tried to talk to Don's kids, but they were met with hostility. Don's friends called regularly; my friends supported me completely; my business clients offered financial help, patience, and flexibility; and my family loved me. They all prayed for me. They would all listen and say, "I don't know what to say. I am just so sorry."

Most of our friends came into our marriage with Don. There were lifelong friends with whom he had gone to college. Our closest friends, the Wrights, were also in real estate, and Gary Wright and Don had encouraged each other through the years. Gary went to see Don at Kate's and found him confused, but seemingly well. Don said to him, "I'd like to find someone to marry if anyone would have me." My husband did not even remember he had a wife who was grieving for him.

February 11, 2007

I am lost. I am nobody. I am invisible. I am somebody else, living someone else's life. I don't even know the person I was. My life feels disjointed and without reality. Like I have been many different people over the years—each with a different life. There's no sense to any of it. (from my journal)

I had worked at a client's office on Wednesday, February 21. It was a beautiful, unseasonably spring-like day, warm and sunny. Don had been gone ten days. I could stand it no longer. I had to see Don or, at the very least, talk to someone, anyone who would tell me what was happening to us. I called often but was answered with a weary, disgusted "What do you want?" and "No!" I knew where

Don was living ... I had sold the house to Don's daughter and her family a few years earlier. I had spent Christmases there; family dinners; birthday parties. How would I not be welcome? I drove over to Kate's home, not far from my own, and rang the doorbell. No one answered, but I could hear the dog and assumed someone was home. In frustration, I rang it several times and then sat down on the front steps *without saying a word*. I wasn't hiding; my car was in the driveway; and I couldn't have appeared threatening, my purse and phone were in the car. It was almost five o'clock and I thought, "Someone will come home soon and talk with me. If it's Larry, he will tell me the truth." I sat there alone in the silence, with the warm sun on my face. I sat on the last step of the porch and drew lines in the dormant dirt of the flower bed as I thought, *I just want to see my husband. I want to know if he is all right. I want to know why you took him from me. I want to know what I have done to bring this action. I just want someone to talk to me.*

Just before five o'clock, two police cars sped up to the house, and two city police officers converged on me. It was impossible for me to take in what was happening. I thought, *This is a terrible mistake!* They ordered me, "Get off the steps!" I could not understand why. I said, "But I'm the *grandmother!*" as though that would explain all. They had their hands on their holsters, and I could see they were very serious! I asked what I had done, and they said I was "*terrorizing*" the family! What madness had this come to? Then Larry's car screeched to a stop sideways in the street; he leapt from his car and, like a bull, ran toward me. The policeman stopped him, but he was flailing his arms and screaming for me to "get out!" He screamed these words: "*She's being divorced*! Her husband doesn't want to see her! He is sick and is in Oklahoma getting treatment!" (In fact, he was in Oklahoma with the girls picking up a $50,000 check.) The police officers then took up the mantra and called me "the soon-to-be ex-wife"! I was weeping and in shock. The neighbors had congregated. I said, "But I know nothing of this! Can't I explain?" But they would not let me speak. They told me to leave without a word or they would arrest me. They said not to ever call there again, or come there again, or I would be trespassing and would be arrested. They took down my driver's license information to make a report, and I got in my car and left. This incident would later be reported in writing that Don's "ex-wife" had come to where Don was staying and "demanded" to see him. Could this get any more absurd?

Our granddaughter, who had spent so many nights at our home, was inside the house and had called the police on me, at the bidding of her father, Larry. At that moment, these people were no longer my children, and their children were not my grandchildren.

I drove away from Kate's house as if in slow motion. I pulled into a vacant lot nearby and tried to recover from the shock. What had happened was incredible. I felt like laughing, but tears came instead. I called my son, Rob—like making a call after a car wreck, seeking someone to confirm that you are still alive and the damage is repairable. I lost track of time as I sat in that empty lot until I felt steady enough to drive the rest of the way home.

So I was being divorced!

That's something you really don't want to hear screamed across the neighborhood. The next day, I talked to a divorce attorney. What was I to do? How could I protect myself against these people? What do I need to protect? Are they using Don as a pawn, or is he doing this willingly? This reeked of James, Carla's husband, the attorney. I always knew he was an opportunist and was neither for nor against anyone; he was in it for the game. But this game was at my expense. Dealing against someone who knows the loopholes of the law and has chosen to make a game of you is very daunting. At my attorney's office, the law partner, whose name is on the building and whose expertise is divorce, told me the best thing for me would be to file for divorce myself—it would be a "race to the courthouse," because the first one to file apparently is in favor. My answer to that was adamant: "I will not divorce my husband." I felt glued to my home, hiding from the mailman as I waited for the divorce papers, or for them to be served by a police officer. I felt like I was being stalked; as though I was in constant danger; as though someone was going to deliver a devastating blow at any moment. I watched every car that passed to see if it would stop and someone would come to my door, delivering another package of devastation. I was afraid one of the kids would try to come into the house and take what they wanted. They had done this to our bank accounts, so I believed they would just take whatever they could get access to. I was afraid to stay home, and I was afraid to leave the house. But mostly I was devastated at the thought of my husband, whom I loved, wanting to divorce me, and I hid behind the doors as though that could keep it from happening. I was paralyzed. The anxiety of the waiting was agonizing.

A week went by and no papers came. On Saturday, Don called me. I thought I was going to faint with relief just to hear his voice. A grown, middle-aged woman still going weak at the voice of her lover! He asked me how I was doing; was I still working? He said he missed me and loved me. But he had heard "through my women's circle" that I had been *poisoning* him. He said he just couldn't live any longer being afraid to go to sleep at night.

Where do these lies come from? How could anyone believe or try to make Don believe such madness? Of course, I told him none of it was true. He told me he had not wanted to believe it but that is what he was told. He asked me to write him a letter saying that it was not true so he could "get things straight in his mind," and he asked for a picture of me. I promised to write him that night. I asked him, "Don, do you want a divorce from me?" "No," he said, "But that is what is happening. *We have to do what Carla says.*"

I sent the letter, which I do not believe Kate ever delivered to Don.

> *February 28, 2007*
>
> *I have been drowning for weeks now. I have not seen my husband for seventeen days. The roller coaster of despair, grief, anger, fear, and frustration has made me physically ill. I have been trying to find some sense in this; a reason, even if it's a wrong reason. Even the wrong reasons make no sense.*
>
> *I have my moments of inconsolable grief. What have I done to these people that they could hate me so much— and hurt their father so much? For a full week they*

have told me a divorce is pending, yet no papers come. This is a cruel game for which I am ill-equipped. (from my journal)

A Moment of Clarity

I lost twenty pounds in the first two weeks, fifteen more in the weeks that followed. I didn't notice. I was grieving the loss of my husband, as surely as if he had died. For me, he had. While I sat every night in our home alone, thinking only of him, he must not have been thinking of me, because he did not call. Had he loved me as I loved him, had he missed me as I missed him, had he wanted to hear my voice, he could have called anytime. But he didn't. So I believed that he did not love me; that he did not miss me; that he did not want to hear my voice; that he was happy where he was; and that it would remain so. I was inconsolable.

The uninvited picture of Don with Kate, her husband and children, and Carla and James sitting around talking and laughing every night together hung in my mind—while I sat alone in our home, grieving. What could they possibly be thinking I was doing every night with Don gone? Most likely they just did not think of me at all.

On the evening of March 6, Don called. He wanted to talk to me; he wanted to see me; he wanted to "make things right between us." He wanted me to come get him. I couldn't make him understand that I could not come there. But then … he didn't know where he was. He said he thought he was in a neighboring town, staying with a couple he didn't know. I knew he was at Kate's, and when I heard Kate enter the room where Don was, I asked to speak to her. She was not happy that he had made the call, was curt, and said she would talk to Don and call me back.

I was surprised when her call came. She said Don wanted to come home to me, and *they would bring him the next morning*. I was like a schoolgirl getting ready for a big date! I laughed at myself as I started planning what I would wear. I cancelled my appointments for Tuesday and waited anxiously for Don to come home.

At the time they were to arrive, I received a call from Doug instead. He said they were not bringing him. He said he would bring Don to *see* me the coming weekend. I had a living, talking person on the other line, and I wanted answers so badly. I put my disappointment of Don not coming home aside and began to ask questions, praying Doug would answer. I asked him the big question: "Why?" After a long pause he said, "*To get a different diagnosis.*" I was astonished. I asked him why that excluded me, and after a long pause, Doug said I had caused Don too much "stress." They were keeping him away from me to avoid stress? I asked, "Is Don filing for divorce, Doug?" Doug stammered a second and then quietly said, "No." "Why did Larry shout that to me and the police that day?" "Well, it was a very stressful situation," he said, indicating that he just couldn't help himself. I said, "Stressful for whom?" and Doug answered, "*For Larry*"!

Was I never to know the truth of why these people took my husband from me?

Two days later, on Thursday, March 8, Don called me around 8 am. He said he was coming home. He seemed to be completely normal, sane, and determined. Like a loose light bulb, his damaged nerve cells would connect at times, and fail at other times. This day, his bulb seemed to be burning brightly. He asked me to come get him, and again I tried to explain that I could not. He said, "I will be home by noon." Almost immediately, Kate called me and said Don wanted to come home, so as soon as they could get his things together they would bring him home. Again, I was stunned. I was afraid to hope for this. Had they tired of him? Had he become too much of a burden? Had he improved? At one o'clock, the car drove up and Don ran to me. He was back. I wasn't sure whether to believe it or not … maybe they had a bungee cord tied to him! They came in with his possessions and sat them down. Carla did not speak or look at me, never removing her sunglasses, but Kate acted as though Don had been out for ice cream and nothing at all unusual had happened. She said I needed to call them when I needed help and added cheerily, "That was what has been missing." I stood dumbfounded!

Don was completely clear. He asked me why I had left him. He said he thought we must have had a terrible fight and that I didn't want him anymore. What kind of cruelty were his children inflicting upon this man? He was stunned and so sorry when I told him what I could of the truth. It seemed clear to him that he was betrayed by his kids, and that they had hurt us both deeply. He was angry with them and did not want to see or talk to any of them should they call. And they did. They called, and they called, and they called. The phone was in front of Don, but he would not answer. I decided that I should contact Don's kids and explain why he was not willing to pick up the phone, and I did so in an e-mail to Kate. This was more than I ever got from any of them when I wanted to talk to my husband. For my trouble, I received an answer that said, in part, "Please seek psychological help for yourself. I'm very concerned about your psychological well-being."

For the next couple of days, we honeymooned. We were alone in our home with each other, and we shut the world out. We just wanted to be together and to love each other. It was so easy to go to sleep at night thinking that we had been restored. It was as if Don had been healed, and our life would resume as it had been. I had been given the gift of "one more day" with the man I loved and had thought was gone forever.

Friday afternoon, our attorney came to our home and visited with Don about his desires and intentions. Don revoked the powers of attorney given to Carla and Kate, and signed medical and financial durable powers of attorney over to me. He said he wanted to make sure this could never happen again. Lying together, he would tell me stories of being at Kate's house that I dared not believe. Much of the time over the past weeks, he was not in reality. I did not want to believe his stories about them any more than I wanted them to believe what he must have said about me. He told me drug dealing was going on, which I dismissed without any thought. He said he had no bed at Kate's and had slept for a month in a recliner. Among his many stories, he told me that the girls had taken him to a nursing home, but he had escaped! He was very detailed about it. He told me about the place where he was, and how upset he was to be there, and how he had run out the front door. I pretty much dismissed that story as well, along with many others. Don asked me to promise him I would never take him to such a place, but would always keep him with me. I made that promise with every intention of keeping it.

The Cuckoo's Nest

By Friday night, Don was becoming sick again. This seemed to be a physical illness; he still seemed to be mentally clear. The month that the girls had him, I had no idea what they had done medically—what doctors they were seeing, and what changes those doctors had made. Kate gave me a list of the medications he was now on, but they had been changed only a day before he was brought home. He had been taken off of his antidepressant and antianxiety drugs (Effexor and Xanax) cold turkey. And now he was experiencing pain and unbearable agitation. He could not sit or lie down. His back, his legs, everything hurt. I tried to call the new doctor whose name was listed, but there was no call back. His old doctors had been removed from his care and could not consult with me. I didn't know where to turn. On Saturday, I continued my calls to the new doctor. Finally an associate called me back and said that it sounded like a urinary tract infection or electrolyte imbalance. The associate advised me that since it was a weekend, I needed to take Don to the hospital, where a doctor would meet us and take the necessary tests. Don had to be in bad shape to consent to the hospital, but he was ready to go. We arrived at the hospital and asked for the doctor. They asked me if Don had ever been treated there before, and I answered no. But then his name popped up on the computer, and they said he had been admitted February 27 and 28. I said no, that could not be. Then the woman looked at me and asked who I was. When I said I was his wife, she said the records showed we were separated. That word hit me like a blow from behind. They told me the doctor was on his way, but soon they put Don in a wheelchair and took us up on the elevator. When the doors opened on the sixth floor, Don panicked. He said he wasn't going there—*this is where he was when he ran away*! I felt like I had ushered him into his worst nightmare! What had I done by bringing him here?

The ward was like the insane asylum in *One Flew Over the Cuckoo's Nest*. The rooms were sparse and had no moving air, no TV, and no towels or washcloths. This was the psych ward. It became obvious that the intent was to admit Don for longer than a urine and blood test. I objected and told the doctor that we were not admitting him. They tried to get Don into a gown and into bed, but he refused to even sit on the edge of the bed. They placated us, as though we were both demented, and left us alone in the sparse, hot room. He paced up and down the hall. I became panicky myself and wanted to run out the front door, too. How could we be in this place? How could this have happened that they would bring him here and not tell me? What had happened here that made Don run away, if in fact he had?

He had.

The staff was well aware by now that Don had left the hospital against medical advice (AMA) a few weeks prior. Now they wanted to make sure it didn't happen again, and they were determined that they were going to keep him at least through the weekend until the same psychiatrists could see him on Monday. They wanted to run the same tests again. I would not let this happen. We came in for urine and blood tests, and by God that's what we were going to get. Hours had passed with no tests. We waited in the hot sparse room or paced the halls. I finally made a scene, demanding to get the two samples taken. A nurse finally came in to take the blood sample, and then after awhile, another took the urine specimen. She looked at it, said it wasn't a sufficient amount, and to my amazement, flushed it away. I wondered how long it would be now until Don could produce a "sufficient amount". After another row with the nurses, another urine sample was taken, and we were instructed to wait for results. Time passed with no communication. We had been in the hospital most of the day. It was now evening. I felt we were being manipulated to stay until Don would be forced to be admitted. I told them we were leaving and they could call us when the results of the tests came in. The nurses stood in front of us and locked the doors to the ward. This had become a *very* bad movie that I did not want to be in. Don was becoming increasingly upset and was beginning to experience evening delirium, when I demanded that they let us go. I knew Don would get so upset that he would become uncontrollable and violent, and then they would restrain him and there would be nothing I could do. I said, "I believe we are still in America," and I took my cell phone and dialed 911. They let us out and wrote "AMA" again on Don's chart.

We were both spent and frightened, and Don was still in pain. I called my personal doctor at 10:00 that night, who told me what to do that might help, and indeed we were able to make it through the night. On Monday morning, we went back to Don's original primary physician. I felt as though we were starting at the beginning again. We had to get someone who would help him and get him back on a medication plan. The neurologist was called back in.

We came home to find a certified letter notice. For some reason I wasn't sure of, Don thought it was divorce papers—coming from his kids to me. He was terribly upset over that notice until we picked up the letter. It was from Frank, making accusations, threats, and ultimatums about the Quarry again. I gave a copy of the letter to Doug, hoping he would step in and handle Frank. But he tossed it aside and said, "That's just Frank," as though we should pay him no mind whatsoever.

On March 18, Doug wanted to come over, bring his sisters, and "talk." He said we needed to "vent." I had bigger things to take care of, but I needed their help, so I told them to come over. They did, bringing grandkids and food as though we were having a freakin' party! Even now, they didn't seem to get what was happening. Don was sick. He had not slept and he was in pain. He could not sit still. He asked them to leave. By midafternoon, I was despairing. He had to have help. I was thinking that he might be experiencing a withdrawal from the medications of which he had been taken off. I called Kate midafternoon and told her I thought we needed to go to the hospital, but I was not taking him to the Cuckoo's Nest! She came, put him in her car, and I followed them to St. Francis Hospital.

At the hospital, they didn't seem to know what to do for him. He was extremely agitated and had severe pain in his back and legs. They gave him Ativan to calm him and wanted to keep him overnight. I was thankful. Carla joined Kate and me about the time he was taken to his room. Because he had had heart surgery, he was put in the cardiac ward. That's a completely different set of symptoms and care level than he required. Before even reaching his bed, he had a fierce, violent reaction to the Ativan. He started ripping off his gown, pulling out his tubes and lines, and hitting or pushing everyone and everything out of his way. He seemed to have the strength of a bull. He grabbed my arm and twisted it and squeezed so hard that I cried out. It was frightening and chaotic. Kate and Carla were both hovering over him, and he was hysterical. The doctor was trying to ask questions, and there were three answers at once. I said, "We need one person to answer, and that would be me!" Carla straightened up and said, with pure hatred, "You know it all, don't you? I'm leaving."

I was glad. I needed Kate to go with her. While the nurses tried to get control of Don, Carla, who is a much larger woman than me, stood in front of me and said, "I have all his money and you are not getting it!" I felt her hatred as if it were cold air spewing from an open freezer. I was in no mood for sass. In the movies, the comeback is something clever and scene stopping. All I managed to say was, "I should slap your stupid face." I will never get her response out of my head. She smirked at me while she gingerly sipped a coke and said, "Go ahead. Slap me. I want you to." I asked the doctor to have her removed, and after she refused to go, security threw her out. The nurses took over Don's security, moving him to a private room, removing him from the patient roster, and giving me a password so only I could see him or inquire about him. I absolutely did not request this action. The nursing staff was not going to allow another fiasco like Carla had just caused.

To me this seemed to be the onset of a very bad war between Carla and me, but now I can see that it had been brewing in Carla for a long time.

That night in the hospital was torture. Don could not rest. He ran up and down the halls, dragging me behind him, until I couldn't walk anymore. He tried to get on every elevator and run out of every door. His feet became blistered and sore. He was exhausted, but could not stop. He was finally given something strong enough to put him to sleep, and I went home to shower and rest. I was back in a couple of hours, only to find Don up running the halls again. This time he was being accompanied by two security guards instead of me. By morning, the hospital had called in psychiatrists, social workers, and his neurologist. Don answered the standard dementia questions of date, year, place, and name, failing miserably, and bought himself a one-way ticket to Prairie View Rehabilitation Hospital in Newton for observation and evaluation. He had totally lost contact with reality. I just hid my face when he told the doctors he was in Russia and that he trained dogs for a living. In a fit of anger and frustration, he told me I was his enemy and that he did not want to see me again, and he pushed me away. This time, the rejection came from him, and I could not bear it. With no sleep and the trauma of the last few days, I was broken. I could stand anything except my husband's rejection. I sat in the waiting room, sobbing uncontrollably. A nun and several social workers tried to console me, one by one, but there was no consolation for me on that day. A cold rain was falling when they put him in a transport and took him away again in the dead of night.

I had tried to call Kate before signing the papers to have him taken to Newton, and after no response, I tried to call Doug in Dallas. No response. I felt guilty for committing him, which I promised him I would never do. Instead of his children, I had to turn to our friends the Wrights for help in making this terrible decision.

On that cold, rainy night when I arrived home from the hospital, weary after two days straight, there was a card in the door and a message on my phone. I had been visited by the Adult Protective Service division of the SRS. I had been reported as being both verbally and physically abusive to my husband and accused of stealing his money for my personal gain, and to be sure, they would be back to investigate me.

In her anger, Carla had made this false report, but I now had to deal with it.

I could not stand any more rejection from Don. I was relieved to be out of hell, if only temporarily. I assumed that Prairie View would not want visitors until they got the patient settled in and I was content to give it some time. I thought I might never visit him at all. But on the second day, I simply stood up in the middle of a meeting and quietly left my clients and drove to Newton. When I got there, Don ran to me when he saw me. The staff said he would not bathe or brush or sleep. When I spoke to him, he calmed down. I took him immediately into his room, where we both undressed and got into the big handicapped shower together. I bathed him thoroughly, washed his hair, and brushed his teeth. And then we lay down on his small bed together and he slept. This became our routine every day. The doctors and nurses said they looked forward to the care I gave Don and to the calmness I brought to him. (Later Don's family would accuse me of being "indecent" with him by showering him.) Here he was diagnosed with *Lewy body dementia, with a side order of adjustment disorder with mixed anxiety and depressed mood, cognitive disorder and panic disorder, psychotic disorder, delusional disorder, aphasia (inability to form words), prosopagnosia (face blindness), and dissociative disorder.* Although someone went over the release papers with me, I don't think anyone ever discussed the reality of his condition with me or explained what these strange words meant to us. Occasionally, Don would act out and be aggressive and even violent. He had physically attacked a doctor once and they put him out with Haldol for twenty-four hours. When he woke up, he was fully rested and seemed much better. At the facility, he could not sleep, pacing and running all night long. Sleep deprivation was becoming a large part of his problem. I had no idea how bad the effects of sleep deprivation could be, but I was soon to find out.

There was a strange phenomenon with Don; although he could barely walk at times, had no depth perception, and appeared very weak, he could go to the basketball court and shoot hoops for long periods. I told the doctors about this and they actually took him to the gym in the facility and watched him as he played on the court. No one could explain it, least of all me.

After two weeks at Newton, the day I took him home he was clear and happy. We stopped at a restaurant and ate a big breakfast. At home, he still suffered from the leg pain, agitation, and inability to sleep. He was on many medications, and the doctors were experimenting with Sinemet, a form of dopamine for Parkinson's, and Seroquel, a form of sedative. They kept increasing his dosages, but still he did not sleep. He began to walk crookedly, and he had extreme pain in his legs. He could not get into or out of the bed without help. We devised our own way to get him in and out of bed by seating him on the bed and then lifting his legs and turning his body. Don is a large man, and I am a small woman. This was difficult for both of us, and it took its toll on us both.

It was heartbreaking to watch Don suffer. I could hear his brother's voice "Help me, Donnie, help me."

How Much Worse Can It Get?

Another doctor, another MRI, and then cortisone shots for a bulged disc. The cortisone made a positive difference. Don's body straightened up, and he could get in and out of bed again. I was desperate to put in a full day's work. It was almost April 15, and none of my client's work was ready for taxes. I had made formal pleas to Carla for the money they had taken so that I could put Don in day care. Without help, it was virtually impossible for me to work. They simply refused to return the money, and I got no help through the legal system. They said they were still holding it for Don's care. I researched nursing homes, knowing that it was inevitable and could not be put off much longer.

The very thought of a nursing home has always made me feel terrible, believing it was a fearful place to be. Knowing nothing of dementia or long-term end-of-life needs, I had many misconceptions of these homes. In recent years, the nursing home concept has changed. Single-family homes are being renovated to accommodate four to eight people in a home-like environment. They have the same caretakers every day, and they have free run of the home; it *is* their home. Meals are home cooked, and the residents usually have lovely and secure yards where they can walk or sit freely. And yet they are full-care nursing homes. I found one such home for Don, Byron Cottage, within walking distance of our home. I imagined walks with Don and even visits to our own home together. Don's children visited the Byron Cottage and approved it.

When Carla received the first month's bill, she refused to pay it. I was sucker-punched yet again! I could not pay $5,000 per month while they held our money! They would not participate with the money of ours that they had taken unless I signed a HIPAA authorization they sent me, which I considered no more than blackmail. In part it read:

> I, Carol (Pendergrass), acting as POA for (my husband), hereby voluntarily waive any physician-patient, psychiatrist-patient, dentist, healthcare professional, or provider privilege to privacy that may exist in my favor and I authorize **my** examination by physicians and psychiatrists and authorize their disclosure of **my** physical or mental condition to **my** personal representatives" (all five of Don's children). (Bold emphasis mine.)

If taken as written (and it is a legal document), I was not only giving up Don's rights but I would be giving his children access to my personal medical information. I was incensed by what I thought they were asking me to agree to and tore the paper in shreds and mailed it back to Carla in her self-addressed, stamped envelope. I would find a way to pay for the care Don needed without the stolen money, which meant I would probably have to borrow it since I could not sell any of our assets due to the demands on the properties by Don's kids.

I needed the day care that Byron Cottage could provide. I thought it would be the answer to me being able to work. I could afford to pay for day care a few days a week myself. At home, Don would not let me out of his sight, and he was jealous of whatever I did. I could work about five minutes before he began to make demands. We went to the day care. He refused to get out of the car, calling me a liar and a trickster. He physically fought the caregivers and me, at times violently, hitting and punching. Once he knocked me out of the way and fled, running down the road. I was beginning to feel that I had no options.

Finally, I found a certified nurse's assistant (CNA) to come to our home to take care of Don while I worked. He didn't like Sherry, but he didn't like me at that time either! He became verbally abusive and, in his misery and psychosis, called us both names I had never heard on his lips. He knocked food and water out of our hands. He spit his food or medications across the room. He physically fought against Sherry and me constantly. He would simply refuse to sit or lie down or cooperate in any way. He refused to put on clothing. He paced, and he ran. He pushed furniture around, and he pulled a large cabinet down on top of himself. He would get so exhausted that he would fall asleep standing up and eventually would fall down. He could not be forced to do anything. He was strong and could outmaneuver anything we tried faster than we could react. It took both of us full time to tend to him.

Show Me the Money

Our attorneys were talking to each other, but little was getting done. My attorney wanted to "settle" with the kids, but I couldn't imagine what that meant! What were we settling on? What were we settling with? I still did not know what they wanted from me.

Doug was again in town from Dallas. Doug is a successful corporate attorney whose job involves mediation and negotiation. Doug is most like Don in his looks and ways, but he is sullen and reserved. Doug was always calm and intellectual, and I respected him. I felt through this ordeal that if any sanity came to this situation, it would come from Doug. Doug wanted to meet with our attorney and Don and me, and I agreed, thinking this meeting might bring reason back into the situation. The following is what Doug said Don's children wanted from me, in part:

1. They would let me take care of Don on a daily basis.
2. Kate and Carla would have Don's medical POA (which means they make all the medical decisions to the exclusion of me).
3. Doug would hold conservancy (financial POA) over all of all our money and our assets.

These three things bespoke our future. They would allow Don to stay with me if they had control over him and our finances. I was being demoted simply to "caretaker." Don's children wanted our marriage to simply not exist, since they were unsuccessful with a divorce. Our friends said the obvious: "It's about the money!" But I refused to believe that. We didn't have that much, and they were all more financially secure than us! It just didn't make sense. But ... what did?

I was incensed that they would think me incapable of handling our finances after sixteen years of marriage! I was entrusted with the administration of my client's multimillion-dollar estates, but could not handle my own finances? I refused to discuss it any further. They were strangers stepping into our financial lives where they had no right to be. There were words between Doug and me, as Don sat silently between us. I would listen to no more and left the room. Later Don smiled at me and said, "You have such spunk! That's what I love about you the most." I accepted that compliment with mixed feelings. I was glad I hadn't disappointed him, but damn, I wished he would speak up for me just once!

It was apparent that Frank, the Sacred Cow, had heard a skewed rendition of our situation and believed that our marriage had broken up. Once again he wrote a threatening letter saying he was forcing *me* to sell the Quarry. This was one thing I was not going to deal with. But within a few weeks, he filed a lawsuit against us, demanding that the Quarry be sold on the courthouse steps. He claimed ownership and expected to receive a portion (to be determined by the court) of the sale price. *This was a joke*, I thought. Being a real estate agent, I knew the law was clear on real estate: if it isn't in writing, it doesn't exist. So I gave little thought that this was serious. Surely the law was on our side.

I still had not learned my lesson about our legal system.

The Sun Goes Down

I hated for evening to come. In late afternoon, Don would begin what is known commonly as "sundowning"—evening delirium. His mood would change, and he would either get very depressed or very agitated. And he would not sleep, although he was exhausted. He would lie down for ten minutes or less, and then he was up again, pacing, running. He couldn't tolerate the darkness, so every light in the house was on all night long. He again became unable to get into or out of bed by himself, so every time he got up, I had to help him out of the bed. Then back into bed ... for a few minutes. All night long. Eventually, neither of us slept at all.

Cleanliness became a thing of the past. If he would consent to a shower, he would sit down in the shower, and I could not get him up. There were times when, through my tears, I had to ask the neighbors to help me get him off the shower floor. He was too aggressive for me to bathe, and he was unable to take care of himself.

He became wild; completely unpredictable. Then he started threatening me. I would wake up to him standing over me with a wild look on his face, saying, "You need to be shot between the eyes." He would ask me if I had ever been hit upside the head with a two-by-four. For no reason, he would grit his teeth in uncontrollable anger and lunge at me. Don would actually laugh as he came after me. He would catch my arm or leg in his arm and twist until I was off the floor. At times, I had to barricade myself from him until he calmed down. I started sleeping on the couch in the living room, where I could see his every move and he couldn't sneak up on me. At night from the couch, I would watch him almost run through the house, back and forth, talking to his friends (who were not there). He would go into the kitchen and stand at the counter as though working intently on something, talking to himself. All night, he worked. I would wake up to find the rugs rolled up and hidden. The sheets were off the bed and in the shower. He pulled the plants apart. He wrote on the kitchen counters with pens and markers. He tore the light fixture down above our bed and it shattered where we would have been sleeping. He would turn the oven broiler on or throw the dishes in the trash. I tried to keep a journal of our nighttime activities but after twenty minutes, I had been up and down so many times I could not keep up with it. Sleep deprivation was fast becoming our worst enemy. I can see why it is used as an effective form of torture.

Where were the doctors during this time? No one seemed to want to be involved anymore because of the familial circumstances. Don absolutely refused to go to appointments I did make, and Sherry and I together could not force him to get dressed and into the car. He seemed too ill for appointments; and after the stay in Prairie View, where was I to take him? I telephoned his doctors often, and they would tell me to up dosages or prescribe a new medicine.

And then Don became incontinent.

Adult Protective Services paid us a surprise visit the morning of April 3. As soon as I opened the door, the lady handed me her card and pushed her way past me to the bedroom where Don was and closed the door. Don was not dressed and was still in bed. When she opened the door and joined me in the living room, she informed me that she had examined Don and had talked with him and found absolutely nothing to substantiate Carla's claims. (One of the claims was that Don wanted to divorce me, but he denied this to her and convinced her that our marriage was happy. Thank God!) She questioned me, and when she left she asked, "Why haven't you filed charges against these people yourself?" I answered, "I'm trying to hold a family together." She told me she was going to talk with the SRS attorneys and see if they could bring charges through their department for financial exploitation (because Don's children had taken our money and were keeping it from us). Apparently one of the accusations made against me was that I locked Don in the bedroom. The agent checked my doors and found that our bedroom doors had no locks! She added, "But that *is* what you have to do at times with dementia patients."

She said the investigation was over.

April 7, 2007

Don has become incoherent, paces, agitated, doesn't sleep, and doesn't eat. Sometimes he lays down "to die." He has become combative and abusive to me. He uses curses and says he's going to "put a bullet in my head," or makes other threats. He's very smug and seems amused when he says it. He seems weak, but can grab and hurt me. He sees people constantly and holds conversations with them. He sees snakes and animals everywhere. He becomes "glued" to the floor. He is obsessed with sex. He won't get dressed. He's jealous of anyone I talk to on the phone, and he's rude to anyone who comes to visit. [My sister] was here and he kept coming out without his clothes on and motioned for her to leave. I feel isolated. He refuses to go to day care. (from my journal)

When the girls dropped by, they acted as though they had never betrayed me. When I tried to tell them what was happening, they obviously did not believe me. Doug was coming from Dallas for Easter and Don said, "Let's get together." Kate started planning an Easter party at our house with all the kids and families for Easter Sunday. I told them then and there that I was not preparing the dinner, and I would not be present. It was as though I had said nothing—the party was planned!

April 11, 2007

In just a few months, Don's condition has changed; his children have separated us and betrayed us; stolen our money; set him back medically; and alienated us forever. Don has gone from confusion to deep dementia; from depression to believing he's dying; from early signs of Parkinson's to total immobility at times. I have gone from frustration to despair, and now resignation. Sometimes I think nothing more can hurt me with him. He vacillates between verbal and physical abuse to deep passion for me. He's so afraid I'm going to leave him. And what of the day I have to come home without him? I don't know if there is any more grief left in me. (from my journal)

It was Easter. Doug had arrived from Dallas. Nothing more was said about the Easter party as Don's condition worsened. Don was exhausted and I was exhausted. The pressure of work was heavy. Dennis, the youngest, would not even see his dad. Doug said, "He doesn't handle these things well." He's thirty-eight years old! How do any of us handle these things? I needed to work. I needed to rest. It was clear the kids did not believe me when I told them of Don's condition. I wanted them to know the reality of how he was. I asked Kate if they could take Don to her house for the weekend while Doug was here. I was desperate for the respite, and also I wanted them to see for themselves what they would not believe from me.

I will pick up Dad about 10:30–10:45 am. I want you to know that if Dad is in the state you described in your e-mail this morning, I can't take him.

Kate (via e-mail)

Well, of course he was in the state I described! I wrote back for them just not to bother ... I would take care of him myself, however I could. But my hands were tied! They had our money, and I was no longer capable of caring for him.

Not one of his children tried to contact us in any way from April 8 to April 20.

Tension between Don's children and me was spiraling. We no longer had an open-door policy. After the hospital episode with Carla, she being the central figure in all of the actions against me, I told Kate that Carla was not welcome in the house anymore. She could see Don whenever she wanted, but not in my house. Kate said she understood why I would feel that way. The SRS began to look into the taking of our money and had interviewed me concerning that. At their request, I provided them with thorough documentation. As far as I knew, the kids were being questioned, but I was not the instigator of this action, and I was given no updates or feedback at all.

One day in late April, I had gone to a client's office and left Don in the care of the CNA, Sherry. Kate called me about 3:30 and asked if she could see her father. I began to tell her that he was home with the CNA I had employed to care for him, and she said, "Yes, Sherry. I've met her." I was surprised when she told me she was at our house already and wanted to take Don out for dinner. I told her that was good and dismissed Sherry for the day. When I returned home, not only was Kate with Don in my house, but Carla was there as well. They both knew I had forbidden Carla in the house, but they did not respect that anymore than they respected me. I was offended and simply went downstairs to my office without a word.

I got a call from Sherry later, telling me that when Kate first arrived, she had sat with Don and quizzed him about money. Sherry said Kate had asked her dad, "Do you think we have stolen money from you?" and was writing down the conversation. When Sherry objected to the course of her questioning, she said Kate took Don downstairs to my office, out of her earshot. My office had always been absolutely off limits to everyone because of the nature of my business, and taking Don there caused many suspicions.

The evening of that outing with Kate and Carla, Don became sick to his stomach. During the next week, Sherry and I could not keep up with his physical needs. The messes were unspeakable. He was totally incontinent. I so wanted to call Kate and Carla and tell them their father had a present for them, and let them come see what I had to deal with on an hourly basis. I had to totally pull up carpets and discard them. A few terrible times, I wanted to pick up my purse, get in the car, and run away forever because the mess was too difficult to face. He fought anyone who touched him. He would come after me and I had to barricade myself, sometimes for hours, during the night. He would grip my arm or hand like a pit bull and twist it.

I know this is a horrible thing to tell; it was a horrible thing to experience. You might think it is better suffered alone and the words left unsaid. If you are going through it, I want you to know you are not alone. We are good, sophisticated, educated, spiritual people who are either ill or are caretakers of the ill, and the facts are that these undignified, unthinkable things happen to us, and we need not be ashamed.

I had been conferring with the doctors as Don became more uncontrollable, and I was often on the phone with the Alzheimer's Association for advice and support. Don had had diarrhea for over a week. The doctors finally agreed that Don needed to go to the hospital. They said he may be suffering from an impacted bowel. I was startled and couldn't understand how it could be impacted when he had diarrhea. It was Saturday morning, and Sherry had the day off. I was alone with Don, and he was a madman. How was I to get him to the hospital? I thought I would have to call an ambulance, but that would only traumatize him more. I was afraid, and I did not know what to do. I sat and prayed and wept. At that moment, my brother called and asked if he could stop by. I said, "No, it isn't a good time," but then through my tears I cried, "Yes, I need you."

He was just around the corner when he called. It took both of us to get Don ready to go to the hospital, as he was manically fighting us all the way. We got him out to the car but the two of us could not get him inside the car. At just that moment, my son Rob drove up. All three of us were able to get him in the car. It was these seemingly small day-by-day miracles that made me know that God was with us. He was providing for us. I was never alone. The presence of God was always with me and He was letting me know it in tangible ways.

Don was admitted with a bowel impaction and dehydration. We had taken him to St. Francis, and their records reflected the last stay there. The first thing the caseworker asked was that I not tell his kids he was in the hospital. He was in a semiprivate room, and there was only room for one visitor in Don's side of the room. Don was a fall risk, so padded mats were placed on the floor around his bed. When I was not in the room with him, he was restrained, because he grabbed the nurses and physically fought them, as he had me. The hospital found him too combative to do physical therapy and considered him a risk to himself and others. The days in the hospital ran together, with Don sleeping almost all of the time. They cleared the impaction and soon removed his intravenous lines. They said they had done all they could do in the hospital. He was bedfast and not able to participate at all in his own feeding or care. I made arrangements for him to go to the nursing home on Byron, where he had spent a few days of day care. When the owner of the home came to assess him, she told me, regrettably, that they could not take him. He was a fall risk, and with the family of attorneys who seemed poised to sue, they could not take that risk themselves. No other nursing home would take him because of this same condition. Once again, Don's children had blocked the way. I was running out of options, and Don's family still had all our money. I was expected to take care of Don, but they would not relinquish the money they claimed they were keeping "for Dad's care."

And then I met with the doctor.

Once Don was stabilized, he continued to decline; he was not eating or drinking. After five days, the doctor told me that he thought his system was shutting down, that sometimes the brain just says, "I've had enough." In his opinion, unless Don started eating and taking liquids again, he would not live but a few weeks to a month. I was not prepared for that information. Don had taken on a very serene expression and was calm. They wanted to release him, but no nursing home would take him in the present situation. His doctor wanted him to transfer to the in-hospital hospice facility, but he did not meet their requirement of imminent death. So the doctors, nurses, caseworker, hospice, and I conferred, and it was decided that I would take Don home with Sherry, the CNA, and hospice attending. I had one day to get that set up, and no money to take care of Don. I made a call to my bank to borrow money to live on and pay for Don's care.

Rob, at a moment's notice, was in action. Friday afternoon, Rob got a hospital bed and set up the room in our house for Don, and we took him home Saturday at noon. As I drove him through the familiar covered bridge, thinking he would be happy to finally be home, I asked, "Do you know where we are?" and he answered, with closed eyes, "It doesn't matter." My brother helped me get Don into bed, and Don looked around the room and said, "This motel must be expensive!" and then settled into a semicomatose state.

I was worried about Don's children. Not one of them had called or e-mailed during the week Don was in the hospital, and I had not notified them because of the hospital's request. It never once occurred to me that Don would not go home in better health than when he had been admitted to the hospital. Again, I was on the monkey bars, and I kept groping for the next bar. "Get through today," I said to myself, "and then we'll think about what's next." Now I had to tell these children who loved their father that he was gravely ill.

The hospice people were at my door before we got Don into bed. I was amazed at how quickly they integrated into our situation. The first nurse brought all the medications provided by hospice, even though we had a sufficient supply. By nightfall that first day home, I had been visited by three of their personnel and talked with two different social workers by phone. The hospital had made them well aware of our family situation, and they were planning to take an active part in dealing with Don's children. I wanted to e-mail the children (which had become our manner of conversing, and then only on important matters) immediately, to let them know they should see their father. Two of the sons would have to travel some distance. The social workers wanted to wait until the sons got there, so they could meet with them and explain Don's condition in person. We all thought his children would not believe me, no matter what I said.

But I could not take the chance of Don worsening before they saw him. As soon as Don was settled in bed, I sent an e-mail to his children.

> *Don's condition has continued to worsen and the progression is faster than anyone expected. He has spent a week in the hospital with an impacted colon, has become incontinent, and is having difficulty eating, drinking, and swallowing. After weeks of severe agitation and combativeness, he has settled down to sleeping continually, but is at peace. The doctors feel that his system is shutting down. The doctor at first said the prognosis was "weeks," but he began to take a little food in the last two days, so it could be prolonged, but of course, no one knows. They suggest that you all come see Don if you want to, before his condition gets any worse.*
>
> *I brought him home from the hospital today, with hospice attending.*
>
> *Hospice has arranged for a family meeting, with the hope that all of you can be here at the same time, at your earliest opportunity. You can talk about when that time might be and let me know and hospice will answer all your questions. Let's put all else aside and be here for your dad.*

As usual, they did not seem to believe me. These were not words I made up, nor did I want to hear them myself. They were the words of the doctors, in whom we are to put our trust. All five of the kids received the e-mail on Saturday, but none came until Sunday afternoon. Several of them came at the same time, and I left them alone with their father. Don was sleeping almost all the time, as he had in the hospital. He was still very sick. Sherry and I worked very hard to follow all instructions, keeping him clean and comfortable and seeing that his needs were met. He was on a soft diet and liquids. Even when he awoke in the middle of the night, I would prepare a meal of mashed potatoes and gravy or soup. When the kids came, they wanted to feed him and give him water. I was happy for him to eat anything at any time given by anyone, but they did this with accusations that I was *not* feeding him, that he was being neglected. I walked away when they came and left them totally alone with their father. The room was pleasant and cool and comfortable. We had found that music calmed him, and he rested better with it on. He seemed to be exceptionally sensitive to voices and would get very upset if anyone spoke too loudly to him ... let's face it, we always think ill people are deaf! Unless he was called by name, he would not focus on what was being said. I put a note on the door to speak softly and call him by name. This seemed to rile the children, even though they did not speak to me about it. In fact, they only spoke to me when it was absolutely necessary during their visits.

There's a picture of an old farmer standing in his field that has been ravaged by hail. He says of life, "You are in control ... *until you're not.*"

PART TWO

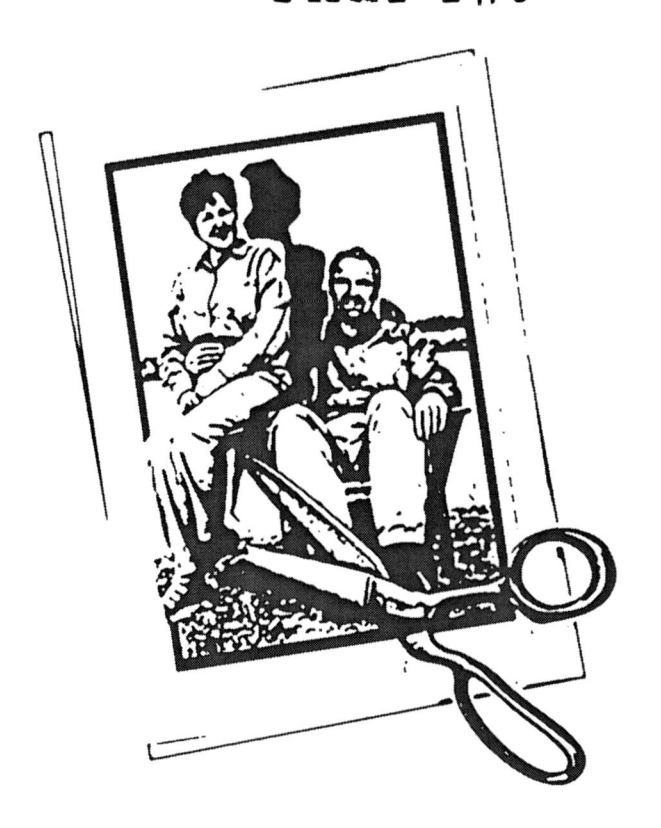

"Surprise!"

Soon I would think of what preceded as "the Good Old Days." Sherry, hospice, or I was always with Don as he lay in his hospital bed in our home. Sherry was there with one purpose: to take care of Don's needs. She was diligent about keeping him clean, dry, and comfortable. Together we fed him and worked on ways to get him to take his medications, which he resisted. We called the nurse or pharmacist to see which pills we could crush up in his food. A lot of the time, he would not swallow and held the medication in his mouth to be spit out later. Every time he opened his eyes, we stuck a spoon in his mouth. He didn't seem to be in any pain; he was weak and in a deep sleep most of the time. He seemed to be gaining some strength. Doug, Carla, and Kate came together on Sunday, Monday, and Tuesday. Tuesday morning, Dale came in from Topeka to see his dad. He was very emotional. He had not seen him for months, so he was having a difficult time making the mental transition from the Dad he remembered to the one lying in a bed, barely conscious. Dennis never did come to see his father.

On Tuesday evening, Don's hospice nurse came by about 6:00 pm. She checked him and said his blood pressure was good, and although he had a very slight temperature, it was to be expected. She checked the intake and outflow records that Sherry diligently kept, and then she left. Our close friends, the Wrights, had come by to see Don and thought he felt chilly to the touch, so I pulled up a light blanket. Doug and Kate came, so I sat in the living room with our friends. As usual, the kids were quiet; they did not so much as give me a nod. Kate seemed to be agitated as soon as she walked in and almost immediately said Don felt hot; she demanded a thermometer. Hot? Cold? Doug went outside to talk on the phone. Then Kate asked for a blood pressure cuff! I didn't have one, and if I had, I wouldn't have known how to use it. She was upset that I was not monitoring his blood pressure. I told her hospice had just left and Don's vitals were all normal. Something was going on with these people, but I could not have imagined what they had already done, and what they were about to do.

The next morning, Wednesday, May 16, four days after bringing him home from the hospital, we got him out of bed, bathed and dressed him, and had him sitting in a chair. That in itself showed significant improvement. It was spring, and the morning was beautiful and sunny. I opened the bedroom window so Don could enjoy the warm, fresh air and the sounds of birds twittering in the big tree outside the window, gathering for their nests.

On that beautiful spring morning, with Don sitting in his chair, I was beginning to feel hopeful again. As I opened the window in Don's room, I saw Carla's van drive up, but she did not get out. I thought about it only for a second, thinking she was probably waiting on Kate. Then Dale's truck pulled up across the street. After a little while, the doorbell rang. I had gone into the bathroom to finish getting dressed and asked Sherry to let the kids in. But Sherry came to the bathroom door and quietly said, "There are policemen at the door!" I thought she was joking—but at the door I was facing four uniformed policemen, Carla, Kate, and Dale.

They filled up the entryway, pushing me back as they forced their way into the house. I could not comprehend what was happening. Kate went directly into Don's room and closed the door. Carla stood in front of me as the older of the officers tried to tell me they had a court order to take Don away. Away? Where? Why? I heard the words, but they did not make any sense. Words cannot express how stunned, confused, and terrified I was. This was madness. Sherry was torn between wanting to help Don and also be there for me.

The officer handed me a document, but I couldn't hold onto it; it slipped to the floor. I told Sherry to call hospice and the Adult Protective Services, and somehow I managed to call my attorney. Almost immediately, the hospice chaplain and social worker arrived. SRS said they had been notified of this action on Monday, May 14! *What?* There was too much to take in.

My attorney said if there was a court order, I had no recourse but to submit.

Sherry called my son, Rob. The house was full of policemen and Don's children. They seemed to take up every inch of space. I was suffocating. Carla stood in my living room in front of me; arms folded across her chest as she blocked my way. She had the same smirk of hate and pleasure on her face as she did in the hospital the night she was thrown out. I thought, "She is enjoying this!" I had no place to go in my own house. I pushed my way around Carla to get out to the back porch. As she blocked my way, I could not stop myself from saying, "I could kill you for what you've done to us." This time she said to the officer standing nearest us, "Oh! She threatened me! You heard it!" I was followed to my own back porch by two policemen and endured a lecture on going to jail for making threats! Threats? Look what they are *doing*! *Is there no sanity in this whole world?*

I ran away from my house and the madness that filled it up and poured out onto my porch, not knowing where to run. I ran across the street to our neighbor's house and nearly collapsed. I had just caught my breath when they told me an ambulance was driving up. Fearing the worst, I ran back across the street to the driveway as the gurney was being taken through the front door. I was barred from even going into my own home.

Someone brought me a lawn chair, and I waited for the dizziness to either pass or claim me. I fell into the chair. I didn't want to live through this moment. My son arrived, and although he was as confused as I, his presence and love comforted me.

The hospice people read to me the ex parte emergency order appointing temporary guardianship and conservatorship of Don to

Kate and Carla. The petition was filed on Monday morning, May 14, two days before, and signed by a judge. In part it read:

> *There is good cause to believe that Donald, the proposed Ward and proposed Conservatee, is an adult with an impairment in need of a Guardian and Conservator, and there is an imminent danger to the physical health of the proposed Ward ... and an imminent danger that the estate of the proposed Ward ... will be depleted.*

That was it. That was all it took to take my husband. No details, no proof, not even an accusation. I did not know what I was being accused of. Surely something concrete had to be offered to the judge that he would take such action. Nothing. Although at the time I could not comprehend it, I did catch the words *guardianship* and *conservatorship* and knew then that once again, these people were robbing me of my husband and my marriage. I heard myself screaming, "How can this happen?"

As this all unfolded, the older officer, who presented me the order in the house, told me how sorry he was to be a part of what was happening. He repeated several times that he had no choice; it was his job. He said to me, "In all the years as an officer of the law, this is the hardest thing I've ever had to do." I believed him.

How I got into the house, I don't remember, but suddenly I panicked and ran to Don's bedroom. One of the officers, a huge man, followed me. Kate was sitting close to Don, and I noticed the shirt Sherry had put on him earlier was now soaked, and somewhere a calm place in my mind wondered what was all over his shirt. Kate told me to get out and shielded Don from me. In the resignation that I would probably never see Don again, I said, "I have to say goodbye to my husband!" She said "No!" and in my desperation, I pulled Kate's arm away from Don. She said to the officer, "She hit me. You saw her hit me." I thought she and Carla must have rehearsed these accusations.

The officer escorted Kate out of the room (out of pity, I suppose), closed the door, and left me alone with my husband, but I knew it was only for a moment. Don was still sitting in the chair in which we had sat him earlier, his eyes closed tightly and his lips pursed. As I put my arms around him and sobbed, he flailed his arms wildly and struck me. I was desperate; I felt I might never see him again. I cried, "Don, do you know what is happening?" He moaned, still with his eyes closed, and said, "Yes." "Is this what you want, to go away with your kids?" I asked, and again he moaned yes while still flailing his arms frantically. He hit me three times, and my heart broke. I kissed him, told him I loved him, and left the room as though I had been beaten nearly to death. I could not bear that our good-bye was to be with that rejection. I thought that would be the last time I would ever see him.

The whole world had gone stark, raving mad.

Alone

As the gurney passed by me in front of our home, Don appeared lifeless. Why were they doing this? Where were they taking him? How much would they put him through? How would he be better off with strangers caring for him than with his wife, in our home? He had just returned from the hospital. I could make no sense of what his kids thought a hospital could do for him when the hospital had just sent him home. Of course, I was told nothing. They said not one word to me. The men with hospice talked to the ambulance personnel and were told that the plan was to take Don to a nursing home. However, when the ambulance arrived, Don's blood pressure began to drop. It became critically low, and that required them to take him to the hospital instead. The hospice chaplain and social worker accompanied the ambulance to the hospital. Later that day, they reported to me that Don had been admitted and that hospice had been terminated.

Out on the driveway, before the ambulance left, I realized I had put the money I had borrowed just days before for Don's care and living expenses in our joint account. I did so in order to give good accounting and so it did not appear that it was being used for anything other than Don's requirements. When I heard the words of the ex parte order, I realized Carla could go straight to the bank and withdraw the borrowed money, and I would be left with that debt also. In my panic, I called the bank to move the money to my personal account and secure it before Carla could get to the bank, as she had done before. Having overheard that panicked telephone conversation with the bank, the hospice social worker saw fit to write it into his report, saying I immediately moved money out of Don's account. Of course, he did not know the details, and I was mortified when I later learned that Carla had received a copy of his report and now claimed I'd "stolen" Don's money. This would come back to haunt me.

I sat in the lawn chair in the driveway. An ambulance, Don's children's vehicles, and four unmarked police cars sped away. Rob, Sherry, and my neighbors stood with me, all of us dumbfounded. The silence was deafening and broken only by my sobs and moans. There were no words that could express my misery and grief, only those mournful sounds coming from my soul. No one knew what to say, because there was nothing to say. Sherry and Rob stayed with me until I asked to be alone. Like an old wounded cat, I wanted to find a safe, dark place and lick my wounds until they healed, or die from them.

I'd been through this separation before. There was no use in trying to contact Don's kids. Now they had a court order, signed by a judge; the ex parte order granted Kate and Carla powers of attorney until a court date could be set for trial. No evidence, no proof. Again, the "law" was a terrible disappointment to me. I was told this judge freely signed such orders upon request with the attitude "It will shake out in the end." I had no right to even inquire about Don's whereabouts or his condition. Should he die, there would be no requirement for them to even notify me.

The lonely days went by. I didn't know what to expect, so I expected nothing. Don had been taken without any of his personal things, not his glasses, not his shoes, not a piece of clothing. The last time I saw him, he was almost comatose. And how had the trauma of all that happened that day affected him? Did he even live through it?

Every day, I searched the obituaries for Don's name. My name. I was inconsolable. The ex parte order alleged that I had mistreated Don and stolen his money. How do you steal your own money? I wanted to refute those accusations. How dare these people take these lies to a court of law? What purpose did they have in this? *What do they want from me?* I didn't even know what the actual accusations were. How can they *legally* separate a husband and wife?

On the streets, I would see couples together, holding hands, driving along, talking. Those sights had a profound effect on me. They were taking for granted that they belonged to each other; that they had a secure place with each other; a husband and a wife; lovers who chose each other out of everyone else in the world to be their companion. Two people who had planned and made a life together in one home. Don and I could have had a child together, old enough to enter college. What if we had had children together? It seemed that the whole world recognized the most basic relationship of marriage ... except my husband's children. I missed my husband and I mourned for our lost time together. He was the most primary person in my life. Tears would fall uncontrollably as I thought how really fragile our lives together are. I forced myself to go out with friends occasionally but I felt that I was missing my reason for even being. The words *How could this happen?* rang in my head constantly.

I was fully expecting to be arrested for assault within a few days. I admit what I said to Carla; although it wasn't a threat, it was a statement and I meant it. And although I did not hit Kate, I wished I had beaten the crap out of her, so I guess you could say there certainly was intent! When the policeman lectured me on my porch, he told me charges could be pressed. I was so defeated that day, I told the officer, "Just cuff me." I was ready to go to jail. Grandma going to jail would make a fine story. I told him, "They've taken my husband from me. I cannot be hurt any more." One of my clients, a wonderful, caring, feisty eighty-five-year-old lady, was so concerned about what was happening to me that she anxiously waited every day to hear every detail of this bizarre tale. When she heard the story of May 16, she was incensed and she told me if they arrested me, my one call should be to her! She was itching to go to the courthouse and post bail, and make sure her opinion of this family was heard! Gladly I accepted her offer, thinking that she had more money than anyone else I knew, and I might very well need every penny of it before this was over.

I no longer looked at the police as the upholders of the law, or as protectors; I no longer saw the law as the seeker of justice, but as the perpetrator of revenge and hatred without allowing me to even be heard. Twice now, I had been accosted by police and not been given an opportunity to even speak for myself, much less seek justice.

How I escaped being charged for assault I'll never know. By now, I knew these people were capable of anything. Maybe it was because they had forced their way into my own home, or maybe the police refused to cooperate. Whatever the reason, it was the only thing they did not pursue! They would not miss another opportunity.

Accusations

The weeks went by. I learned through the attorneys that Don had been admitted back into St. Francis Hospital, where he had just spent over a week. After several days, I got a call from a social worker I had come to know while Don was hospitalized at St. Francis. She said before she was inevitably told that she could not talk to me, she was going to let me know that Don was indeed in the hospital, in about the same condition as when he was there earlier in May. The children were seeking aggressive treatment for him, including physical therapy. The social worker said that had gone badly, and it had made Don aggressive and out of control, as it had when he was in the hospital before, so it was discontinued. She said Don was not listed on the hospital register, which I assumed was in retaliation for the hospital action taken after Carla was banned from there several months ago. I was not supposed to know where Don was. She will never know how I appreciated her consideration of me.

Every day, I got out of my bed expecting to go to war. On May 21, we received the "Details of Petition," which was the document stating the accusations made against me that were to back up the ex parte order. Finally, I thought, I am at least to know of what I am being accused.

The accusations were long and full of "legalese." To summarize, I was accused of "failing to administer medications properly, resulting in [Don] suffering from an impacted bowel ... failing to notify his children of his condition … and [denying] family members access to [Don] and [being] either unable or unwilling to provide adequate care."

The accusations also stated that there was an "imminent danger that the estate will be significantly depleted unless immediate action is taken to protect" it. It read, "His spouse has breached her fiduciary duties by purporting to make unauthorized gifts and engaging in transactions involving self-dealing and/or conflict of interest." I assumed this meant setting up my trust.

So this action was taken because Kate and Carla were accusing me of either overmedicating or undermedicating my husband and causing his illness! And of stealing *our* money. The only truth was that I had put my two personal properties in a trust to protect them from Don's children. I felt relieved when I finally knew these accusations, because I could certainly prove them wrong.

Wasn't it they who stole all the money from our joint accounts? Wasn't it they who denied me access to Don for a whole month?

Oh, well. I was confident that this could be easily dealt with. I could prove that I gave Don exactly what was prescribed by his doctors, and nothing else.

The Electric Chair

On May 25, my attorney received notification that Don's children were now filing a *civil lawsuit* against me. What could this mean? I was terrified. In this letter, we were given notice that my attorney and his firm would be disqualified from representing me in the litigation of the civil suit. They intended to call my attorney as a witness, since it was he who procured Don's powers of attorney for me and drew up my trust papers. I was being forced to find another law firm and start all over with someone new to the case. This was most upsetting to me, since my attorney had been my associate, my friend, and Don's attorney for many years and knew the history of everything involved. Of course, it appeared that was their strategy.

Another firm, another attorney, and the bills kept mounting. I suppose no case is simple, but it seemed insurmountable to bring my new attorney up to date and to explain the family dynamics of the case. He admitted that he did not really believe how bad this was and thought I was exaggerating, until he got deeply involved in the case.

Finally, on June 27, I was served with the civil lawsuit. For a whole month, I had again been terrified every single day of what was coming. When I saw my husband's name as "Plaintiff," suing me, I couldn't believe I was seeing those words. If Don could know what was happening, he would be livid. My new attorney, with whom I had now become well acquainted (I was making monthly payments on his new car!), warned me that I would find the wording of the petition insulting and offensive to read. The petition asserted three distinct claims. Two of them alleged conversion of Don's funds and breach of fiduciary duties owed to Don. The third claim was a *personal injury claim*. They contended that I overmedicated Don and caused severe dehydration. They contended that I had purchased approximately four times the amount of Cymbalta and Seroquel that was prescribed for Don, which they charged I then administered. They were suing for $75,000. This was in addition to wanting all of our assets converted to them for Don's care.

The misinformation included in the wording of the civil suit was astounding. Without proof, they made statements that Don was responsible for our house payments, the truth being that when we bought the house, I had used my inheritance to make the down payment (a third of the price), and for the remainder, I took out a mortgage in my name only; Don had never made a house payment. They erroneously stated that Don was owner of my condo and liable for the mortgage, which again is in my name only—in fact, it is in my maiden name. They laid claim to my personal accounts as belonging to Don, and alleged that I had withdrawn $12,000 of Don's money (the recently borrowed money I put into his account) for my own benefit, saying, "Such withdrawal constituted an act of self-dealing in breach of Carol's fiduciary duties to Don."

The petition went on to say that "Carol obtained prescriptions for Don and directed him to take them, *which he did*. Those prescriptions were sufficient to last Don more than 160 days." Also, "Carol *caused* hospice to deliver painkillers so they could be administered to Don." (Emphasis mine.) I was misquoted several times in the lawsuit, and at the end, it was alleged that Don's diagnosis of "acute renal failure, delirium, dehydration and hypotension [was caused] by being over medicated by Carol and/or her lack of reasonable care of Don." By the time I had read all of that, I could see myself in the electric chair.

I was being accused of trying to murder my husband.

These allegations could be refuted with simple common sense! I didn't prescribe the medications. I gave any medications prescribed as directed. How does one "cause" hospice to deliver medications? To my knowledge, Don had no pain medications. When they first delivered his meds, they left something for *agitation*, but I never used it; the bottle was still sealed. Don showed no indication that he was in pain. Actually, most of the medications were duplicates and had not been opened. I had no knowledge of Don ever having acute renal failure or hypotension. Where were these accusations coming from, and who would believe them? Apparently Don's children were confident the court would believe them, because they asked for an award of "an amount in excess of $75,000 for damages arising from Plaintiff's personal injuries."

How is it that when a father gets sick that the mother is blamed? I tried to sympathize and imagine that these people had never faced the death of a parent before, but they were none of them children anymore, all on the threshold of middle age. My father died of a short illness when I was twenty-nine, and it would never have occurred to me to blame anyone. Is it the mentality of a family of lawyers to lay blame and seek restitution because they know how? The question hung over me constantly why they hated me so much and when did the hatred start. These questions were ones for which I would find no answer.

Maybe they didn't like my Halloween costume last year.

All of our friends sought answers, too. Most of our friends were Don's friends long before I knew Don, and they came with Don to our marriage. They knew us both, and they knew us together. Most people said, "It's the money!" I never believed that because there just wasn't that much of it. Some wondered if Don's ex-wife could be behind this. I thought that possible, but if she were, and I were her new husband, I would be getting out of Dodge! Don's oldest friend from their college days said he believed that many times with a second marriage, the children "go along" with the marriage because they know their relationship with their parent depends on their acceptance of his new mate. But they lie in wait for a moment when they can move in and reclaim their parent for themselves. This was believable. For eighteen years, Don and I both had believed his children accepted me and our marriage. They must have felt that if they failed to accept me, they would lose their father. They knew I made him happy. They were willing to "go along" until the door opened. But nothing really made any sense.

Stand in Line

As the days passed, I spent more and more time in the office of attorneys. Frank's lawsuit over the Quarry escalated. The attorney fees were mounting, and I learned another lesson about the law.

I'm aware that a person can sue over anything—even with no basis, or as a nuisance. It doesn't matter if it defies the law, or sanity. But I thought that the court recognized these nuisance cases and dismissed them as having no validity. What I learned was that once a lawsuit is filed, it must be resolved, either by settlement between the parties or by action of the court. Frank's lawsuit was ludicrous as well as going against real estate law. I guess I thought that once his attorney saw that he had no case, they would have to drop it for lack of anything to substantiate their demands. That's not the way it happens. Both sides have to present "discovery," ours being that the Quarry title is held in a limited liability corporation with Don and me as the only partners. Frank's side was that he and Don had had private conversations giving Frank ownership. He had no witnesses. His claims were laughable. I soon realized I was going to be laughing all the way to the courtroom! Until the lawsuit was legally resolved, a cloud hung over the Quarry title, and I could not sell it. The section it sat on was our nest egg. As that property increased in value over the years, it was to be mine and Don's retirement. And now, when

I needed the money for Don's care, I could not sell it. This family had completely tied my hands financially.

In Frank's lawsuit, the attorneys were talking settlement, which went against any idea of fairness or justice that I had. They were going to try to buy Frank out by offering him cash—a substantial amount. Why should I have to pay him anything? Where is the law in this? The written law is on my side! I am in the right. But because he wants it, I'm going to have to pay him to get off my land? The answer to that is "Yes." A big complication was that I did not know what encouragement the children were giving to Frank, but I was pretty sure it was to benefit him, not Don and me. You know, the old Sacred Cow syndrome.

Once again, I sat at the big table in the conference room of the law firm. Sometimes I wondered how this family could stand each other; how could they live with what they, as a family, were doing to me. Did they not realize that what they did to me, they did to Don? Every day, a new wrench was thrown in my life. I learned they had opened a post office box and any mail with Don's name on it was being forwarded to that box. That meant I was not getting the household bills. I was not getting my bank statements, insurance notices, and so on. I had enrolled in broker's classes and had to cancel because of court or deposition dates they set. Every plan I made was at the mercy of the schedule they set for me. I felt entirely out of control of my life. I pictured them all sitting around a campfire, dreaming up what they were going to do to me next. These sometimes small but time-consuming complications were keeping me from working or living in any measure of peace.

I was desperate to renew my real estate license. Both mine and Don's licenses expired in March 2007, and of course, Don would not be renewing his license. After several attempts to attend classes, I was finally able to take the classes to renew my real estate license. For many years, I anticipated the closing of a large trust that I administered and would have the opportunity to sell $3 million worth of prime pasture land in the Flint Hills of Kansas. That time had come, and I had no broker. I had planned for some time to get my broker's license but as long as Don was my broker, there was no hurry to make a change. Now the pressure was on. Finally, in September, I was able to attend the one-week class, passed the tests, and received my broker's license. I then founded my own real estate company with the sole purpose of making this one sale and recovering my financial stability with the commission.

With the three lawsuits proceeding against me, I had no idea if I would come out with the clothes on my back. I had been ordered to provide tax returns, personal bank account information, appraisals of my home (which I had almost paid off) and my rental home (still in my maiden name), as well as all jointly owned assets. They even demanded a list of all of our household furniture and goods with their respective values! I was sent copies of my personal bank accounts with deposits and withdrawals noted that I was to explain, as though I were somehow pilfering money from Don. The deposits were either my own wages for my business or real estate commissions. The noted withdrawals were for the same amount each month: my house payment. I was offended and enraged that I should have to justify these to my husband's children. Early on in Don's illness I had, against my will, given Doug a complete history of our finances from the date of our marriage, detailing how we managed our finances and assets. Nothing would change from that initial information, even under oath! But they seemed to accept nothing I said, even if I proved it to them.

One issue was that Don's children believed he owned a substantial condominium development. Perhaps, in his dementia, he told them that. But he had no such interest, and never had. Before we were married, he had been a minor partner in a small block of town homes, but the partnership broke up and Don received ownership of *one* of the town homes as his share. Of course, when I explained that to them, the kids did not believe me. It became obvious that they believed that their father was much more successful than the reality of our middle-class existence. Don had come into our marriage with enormous debts on the cattle loss. The money he generated during our marriage went to those debts and into his businesses. His children would not believe that my income sustained us.

And then they demanded all the records of the real estate and management companies. I was summoned to a predeposition inquiry, which took most of the day. I was grilled about every account. It was not I who got these companies into dire shape, but I had done my best for the past year to remedy it. And now I was being accused of misusing the company funds, or of stealing them for my own gain. They wanted to know what I did with the proceeds from the sale of the management company, accusing me of stealing it. They refused to acknowledge our conversations about the sale and the conclusion that there would be no proceeds. I was afraid. But not so afraid that I would not take a stand for myself and express my outrage at these fools. If I am anything, I am a record keeper. I meticulously gathered all my books and documents and was ready to stand my ground against the accusations. I was grilled about every line on my financial records and answered, sometimes through gritted teeth, their insulting questions. Finally, the opposing attorneys came to the accusation of the medications. I was also ready for that.

With as many doctors as Don had seen in the last year, or even months, each one prescribing their own medications and changing the ones from the last doctor, we had accumulated a lot of prescription medications. When Don left St. Francis Hospital, they prescribed medications and I didn't question them, I just filled them and gave them as prescribed. Then hospice brought medications, which they provided without charge, and left them in our home. One doctor prescribed Seroquel, a drug for calming anxiety, in one dosage, and then in half that dose; therefore, we had prescriptions for both dosages. There were many "retired" medications. I had them all in a box to present to the plaintiffs. I had counted every pill in every bottle, and there was no question that the accusations of the medications were completely unfounded. Every pill was accounted for. It was ludicrous to assume that because we were in possession of any certain medication, that I had forced Don to take them in total.

The attorney representing Don's children gave me no slack. He tried to be intimidating. He wore reading glasses down on his nose. He would look up over the glasses with an accusing stare, and all I could see was an old school master from *Oliver Twist* about to whack my hands with his long pointer. The curse to find something funny in almost anything overcame me, and it was all I could do not to laugh as I tried to keep my wits about me. Until the very last moment, he gave no idea of how he received my testimony. His last words to us were that he was going to recommend *a quick settlement to this dispute,* and he was sure his clients would go along with it. We could expect the papers in a few days. My attorney and I thought that the two opposing attorneys felt there was no case to pursue.

When served with the civil lawsuit papers, I was terrified. Could I be charged with manslaughter? Could I be found guilty of causing Don's illnesses? I began to doubt myself. I contacted Don's primary physician, who was the "master mind" behind all of his treatment. He agreed to see me just to discuss Don and my present situation. Of course, he was already aware of much of what was going on, as it was his hospitalist (a doctor on his staff who sees his patients only in the hospital) who told me Don was not likely to live long when we left St. Francis, and it was another of his hospitalists who took over Don's care in the hospital when his children took him there from our home in May. But when I told him I was being accused of causing Don's illnesses, he described those accusations, and the people who were making them, as "despicable." He assured me there was no way that anyone can cause a bowel impaction. He assured me that the diagnosis of Lewy body dementia had not changed. He assured me that he would be willing to testify to that, but he did not believe I could ever be accused of such. He told me Don's situation was so out of control with his children that he was going to write a letter of resignation as Don's primary physician. Whether he carried through on that I do not know; however, I do know that he is no longer Don's physician.

I also talked with Don's neurologist, who had first diagnosed him with Lewy body, and he also assured me that I could not be blamed for any illness and that Don's diagnosis had not changed. Don's psychologist and PA also assured me of the same. The general consensus among the doctors was that I was not a doctor, and I carried out the orders of the doctors and could not be held accountable for a doctor's prescriptions, orders, or diagnosis.

Reunited with My Husband

When the hospital ascertained that Don's acute needs were met, as they had in May with me, he was scheduled to be released. His children apparently had a difficult time finding a nursing home that would take him. For whatever reason, they moved him to a nursing home in Newton, Kansas. Apparently, the first night there he experienced a "catastrophic reaction" and became violent; he was strapped down and taken by ambulance to the psych ward in Newton Hospital. He had been there about a week when I was finally told where he was and that I could see him. I doubt that I would have been told even then where he was, except that Kate had given a list of items, including Don's glasses and items of clothing, that I was to deliver to her attorney. My attorney responded that I would deliver them to Don personally or not at all. I was so anxious to see Don after three weeks that I nearly flew to Newton. I only wanted to be with my husband. I was allotted the hours of 11:00 to 1:00 weekdays by his children to visit my husband of sixteen years. On June 7, I drove to Newton for the first time.

Newton is a small town about forty minutes from our home. Spring was turning to summer, and it was a lovely day. I was so excited to see Don, and I felt strangely young and in love. "How silly," I thought. "I'm going to a geriatric psych ward!" I walked in, wondering if the man who had such passion for me a few months ago would even know me. I had no idea in what condition I would find him; if he would know me, or want me. As soon as Don saw me, joy seemed to come over him, and he hugged me and kissed me and introduced me to everyone in the ward as his wife. I wept with relief to be with him again, and to know that he loved me.

He was confused about why I had been "gone." He wanted to go home with me; why then could I not stay with him? He said he only wanted to be with me, anywhere.

The nurses wondered who I was. Although he had been there a week, they had never been told Don was married, that he had a wife who longed for him, but was being kept from him. In his room was a collage of pictures of his children and grandchildren, but no suggestion of his life-mate. On the wall were the names of his children and their telephone numbers. Conspicuously, mine was not there. Still they try to dismiss me, to take me out of Don's life. I wanted to take red paint and write my name—"WIFE: CAROL"— all over the walls and floors and on the bed sheets. I wanted to tell them that I do exist, and because Don loves me, I am not going to go away!

I realized the possibility that in his present condition, he may live only "in the moment," so that when I was gone from his sight, he may not think of me at all. What more a miracle, then, when I appear out of his yesterdays or tomorrows, he loves me. Though they take away his body from me, these betrayers will not—cannot—take away our love.

The next day, June 8, I could hardly wait to drive back to Newton and be with Don. I wore his wedding band on my thumb so that I could put it once again on his finger. I wanted him and everyone else to know "This man is my husband!" If only a ring on his finger, I wanted his children to have a reminder that they had not been successful in tearing us apart. When I arrived, Don was anxious, sitting in the hallway facing the door, fearful that I would not come. As soon as I arrived, he took my hand and almost ran to his room. He wanted me to lie beside him on the bed. I lifted his once heavy legs onto the bed, and they seemed weightless. As long as I lay still, he slept. If I moved, he would jerk up anxiously. He would not let go of my hand. As we lay quietly together on his bed, he whispered to me that he knew he was in jail, awaiting his punishment. He thought he had done something horrible, although he couldn't comprehend that he could be capable of doing something bad. I assumed he remembered the ambulance and being strapped to a gurney and all the trauma that went with it; he thought he was being taken to jail. He said he was taken by police; maybe he was remembering the day he was taken from our home. He was heartsick and confused about whatever it was he thought he had done. He seemed to have accepted the fact that he had killed someone, and he kept saying he "beheaded" someone, but he could not remember it. The horror of what he was telling me was almost too much to control lying beside him. Of course, in the psych ward, the doors are locked and secured, and it's institutionalized so it wasn't too far a stretch to see it as a jail. He felt he was being tortured at times. No matter how many times I told him he was a good man and had never done anything bad, the pervading "punishment" he felt hung over him.

 I found Don very unkempt when I saw him in the hospital. This very dignified, arrogant man looked neglected and pitiable. I brought scissors and grooming aids to cut his hair, shave his face, clip his nails, and groom him. After I finished, he looked like himself again, except he was very thin. His clothes were ill-fitting and shabby. Apparently, he had been wearing discards from Larry's closet. I brought him new clothes of his own that fit him. I packed up the shabby things and resisted the urge to burn them. I would return these rags to their owners. The day nurse asked many questions about Don's life and interests. She said there had been *no one* there to visit him during her day shift to ask. She said she had not seen Don have another visitor since he'd been there, which was over a week. I was stunned and angry! Apparently, the kids came in the evening—or so I hoped. To keep me away from him and then leave him alone was unthinkable.

 I saw him every day, during my allotted two hours, and I stole time whenever I could. I would call ahead, and if no one was with him, I would drive the forty minutes to Newton to spend a few minutes with him. He would talk quietly of his thoughts, telling me that he would get very upset and be at his wit's end when he'd look up and I would be there and it was like a miracle to him. He constantly asked about money. He was a man who always had cash and the responsibility of supporting others. He was very distressed that he did not have any money in his billfold. It made him feel powerless. I put money in his billfold and broke the rules by making sure he had it in his pocket.

When I went home, I would sit alone, wanting him. He was there alone, wanting me. What can be right about this? What kinds of laws allow a couple to be torn apart like this because the children are full of hate?

He fell several times, once cutting his face badly. He would often just collapse, saying he was dizzy and couldn't see where he was going. He walked as though his feet were numb, unsure when they touched the ground, and he could not perceive depth so he was never sure when to step up or down. He stopped at every line in the carpet or tile and was glued to the floor, trying to determine if it was a step. His hallucinations and delusions were increasing.

The staff told me that Kate and Carla were interviewing for placement in a nursing home. I wanted him back at Byron because it was so near to our home, and he and I both knew the people there. But if I wanted it, it was sure not to happen. I suspected the girls would put him as far from me as they could.

On June 13, I drove to Newton in a summer rainstorm for my allotted two hours. When I arrived, I learned that the girls had come early that morning and moved Don to a nursing facility. I drove back with pelting rain hitting my windshield; or was it my tears? Another separation.

Within a week, my attorney was able to find out where they had taken Don and got papers in place for me to have full access to Don and to his records. This seemed a victory. That week, I finally saw him in his new home.

Is There No Peace Anywhere?

Nancy Reagan's book *The Long Good-Bye* just came out. In interviews, she wept as she told how her husband's decline with Alzheimer's robbed them of their last years together. And the nation wept with her. Lee Woodruff's book *In an Instant* also just came out, about her husband Bob Woodruff's battle with head injury. Lee drew sympathy and admiration for standing by her husband, as a wife should do, when he was near death. She was by his side every minute of every painful day. Even in the fantasy world, the Frog King in *Shrek* was buried and mourned by his wife, the queen. Why am I different? Why is our marriage not recognized and respected by Don's children? How is it that I am robbed of our last years altogether; robbed of being by my husband's side; robbed of burying him?

Don was gone. I tried to go on with my life. I had time to work now, and I had Rob and my grandchildren. I had a huge yard to take care of, and I spent a lot of time feeding the baby ducks and geese that came to the tree for feeding. I had my broker's license, and I had started my own real estate company. I wrote prolifically in my journal because I thought someday even I would not believe this incredible story if I didn't write it down. I bought a new car … well, a three-year-old car, but it was new to me. Don was a Cadillac man, so we had Cadillacs. Grandma cars. Don's son-in-law, Larry, is the service manager for the Cadillac dealer, so we always bought our cars there, and Don always serviced them in Larry's shop. Now that my Cadillac required service and some major work, I decided to trade it off rather than to take it to Larry.

I have always preferred a small car. When Don and I married, I had a new sports car, which he found too small for his large frame … thus the Cadillac. I was also aware of the fact that because our car was in both of our names, the kids could sell it right out from under me. When I found the car I wanted, my stipulation was that they trade straight across so I could not be accused of spending money frivolously. I talked to my attorney and was aggravated at myself as I struggled with the certainty that I would be criticized by Don's children for trading cars, as though I was not entitled to own the car of my choice … because … everything we owned belonged to Don? I bought a Mazda sports car, and it seemed to change my outlook on going out of the house. It made me feel like I wasn't an old lady who had lost control of her life, with a husband dying in a nursing home.

On June 19, I visited Don in his new home for the first time, a facility fifteen miles from our home. It was a brick 1960s house in a nice neighborhood. There are absolutely no identifying marks to the house that would indicate it was anything but a single-family home. In its former life, it had a swimming pool in the back yard, which was filled in and was now a garden with a walk all around it. It was securely fenced so the residents could freely go outside and walk or sit in the garden. Don had his own bedroom. Until I brought a small couch from our home that Don liked to sleep on, there was nothing in his room that was familiar—except the ever-present collage of pictures of his kids and grandkids on the wall. Again, no sign that he had a wife.

All that Don had to wear were the clothes I had taken to him in Newton and a fresh supply of Larry's ill-fitting clothing hanging in the closet. Larry is several inches shorter than Don and quite a few inches wider, and I was embarrassed by how Don looked in Larry's old clothes. Sometimes, it was necessary for Don to change clothes three or four times in one day. I went through his vast array of clothes at home and chose the appropriate pieces for his living situation and filled his closet with nice new clothing. I bought him new jeans, sweats, jackets, and shoes. Again I put the old shabby hand-me-downs in a sack and stashed it with the one from Newton. My husband was going to look as distinguished as possible, whether in a boardroom or a nursing home.

Don was long past the phase of "the Carols" and the confusion with home. He had no concept of time or place, and although he seemed resigned to where he was, he was very sad that he couldn't be home with me. He expected me to take care of him—to rescue him—and there was no way to make him understand that all my power had been taken away. He wanted to go out. On the first day I visited, I asked if I could take him out for lunch and was told, "You are his wife. I can't see why not." We went to Wendy's for a hamburger. He seemed very happy just to have some normalcy to his life. As we passed the condiment sidebar, Don stopped and picked up the entire pump-container of ketchup and carried it to our table. Nothing wrong with that! He was enjoying his lunch out and we didn't run out of ketchup! When I visited the home, I brought him his favorite fountain drinks and snacks, and our visits went well for about a week.

Then one day, I was asked to leave at noon. I was told that family members could not be present during meals because it was a distraction to the patient. My allotted visiting hours were 11:00 to 1:00, and although I rarely ate with him, other visitors as well as I made the mealtime an occasion to interact around the table with all the residents. This change seemed strange, but I just started coming earlier and left when lunch was served. Then I was told I could not bring a fountain drink into the home—it was against the rules. Every day, the rules were changing, but only for me, it seemed. Each day, I was restricted in some new way. When we moved Don's small couch into his room, we had positioned it on the only vacant wall. I came in one day to see the furniture rearranged; the couch was in a straight line with the bedroom door, which opened out to the kitchen. It was now in complete view of anyone and everyone who walked by or sat at the kitchen table. Of course, the implication was obvious; they wanted to have a clear view of me when I was in Don's room. When I asked about it, I was told it gave Don a better view out his window. That week, Don's wedding ring disappeared from his finger. For a week, no one seemed to know where it was. Finally, one of the caretakers handed it to me without explanation.

One day, I got ready to take Don to lunch but the supervisor told me he could not go out because "it was too soon" and he needed more time to acclimate to his surroundings. Hmmm. Of course I was suspicious of what was going on, but I stored it away and waited to see what would happen next. One Saturday, he begged to go out for lunch, and the caregiver told me that his kids had taken him out that week a couple of times, so apparently the time of being "too soon" had passed. When I asked to take him to lunch, I asked the caregiver to check the books to be sure it was okay that I take him, and there was nothing written or any reason for her to question my taking him. So we went to lunch and then had ice cream. I took him back to the home, and he was asleep before I left.

The following week, the supervisor was present at the home, and when I left, she escorted me out. Outside the doors, she told me she "did not appreciate me taking advantage of the situation and taking Don out." Our conversation was very enlightening on both sides, and when I got home, there was a letter from Kate and Carla's attorney stating in less than tactful words the same accusations that came from the supervisor. The letter matter-of-factly stated that I had attempted to take Don out of the home "permanently." Again, I wondered if there was any sanity in this world. Because I wanted this episode to be verified and put into the records, I sent the following letter to the office of the care home, knowing that it would be read by all the staff:

> *July 11, 2007*
>
> *To: Supervisor of CC*
>
> *This letter is to document the happenings of Monday, July 9, 2007, and the conversations between us of that date.*

After spending awhile with Don, on my way out [the Supervisor] walked out with me. Her first words were "I don't appreciate you taking advantage of the situation and taking Don out." I replied that when I asked to take Don to lunch, the caregiver said she thought that would be fine since he had been going out with his kids that week. I asked her if there could be orders prohibiting me, specifically, from taking him because I did not want her to have any conflict over it, and I asked her to check the books. She pulled two books and checked thoroughly and said there was nothing. When we returned, Don was happy and calm, and he was asleep when I passed by the windows.

I told you that the first day I was able to see Don at the home, I had asked the "rules." I was told there basically weren't any rules for families. That first day I was allowed to take Don to lunch. In the weeks that followed I was welcomed at lunch time and was invited to eat with Don (which I rarely did). The following week, I brought a fountain drink, as I had many times before, and was told "no fountain drinks are allowed." The caregiver poured it out.

My son and I brought Don's couch from home to his room and placed it on the only available wall. Then one day the room was rearranged so that the couch was directly in line with the kitchen door. I was told no doors were to be closed.

Then I was asked not to be present during lunch. It was a "rule." I had been given the hours of 11:00 to 1:00 to visit Don by his kids, so this was a bit of a problem—but again, I said nothing and conformed.

The current problem arose because Don's children were taking him out for the day, or afternoon, or lunch regularly, and the caregivers were making sure I knew it. So when Don would expect to go out with me, nothing I could say would make him understand that I was not allowed to take him out. He would get so frustrated with me that I had no recourse in the conversation. He knew he could go out, so I just must not want to go out with him. He would accuse me of having another man in my life. When I asked, I was told the ridiculous lie—by you—that it was "too soon" for him to be out.

On one occasion I didn't know what to say to him as he kept begging, so I thought if one of the "powers that be" told him no, he would accept it. So I took him to the caregiver (others were present, including you) and so as not to give the impression that it was I who was insisting on going out, I said to Don to ask his question of you. He asked to go out with me, and was again told by the caregiver, and you, that it was "too soon." He was accepting and polite as we returned to his room, but when alone, he started begging again. I can go out to eat anytime, any place I want to. It is Don who begs to go out, not me.

These things were adding up to consistent lies that I was being told. It was obvious that these "rules" were being made up by Don's children for me alone. If I asked anything about Don's condition, I was lied to or not answered at all.

I explained to you what you were already fully aware of—that Don's children had filed a very incriminating lawsuit against me. It was apparent by your reaction that you believed me to be a threat to Don. You also told me that "when the SRS completed their investigation" of me, it would be over. I told you I knew nothing of this! The SRS had investigated me at Carla's bidding in April and found me above reproach. Later in the day in a phone conversation you mentioned our "business": you had apparently believed stories about where our money was coming from. The facts are that Don had a real estate brokerage and property management company that basically supported itself as long as Don was involved. When his capacities began to diminish, so did his business. It is from my business our expendable income comes. I mention this only because the information you got from Don's children seemed to affect your perception of the situation.

I called you later when I received a letter from Don's children's attorney accusing me of the same thing you had—upsetting Don and causing anxiety by enticing him to "go out temporarily and permanently." This just adds another accusation to the lawsuit. I spend 75 percent of the time I have with Don trying to say, "No, I cannot take you out." Being able to go at will with his children, but not his wife, is causing Don anxiety, not suggestions from me. Believe me, spending the precious time I have with him trying to find 100 ways to say no is not what I want to do. And as for the "permanently," that is a blatant lie. I was the one who cleaned up after him, never slept, and was the brunt of his combativeness when he was in much worse condition than he is now, and I know I cannot return to that. He is where he needs to be.

Briefly I told you how Don's children had taken Don out of our home—once as though he were being kidnapped, and again after a life-threatening illness, with a court order. They had hidden him away from me for four weeks the first time—without ever explaining why, enticed him to file for divorce, and convinced him I was poisoning him; and it was three weeks the second time that I did not know if he were dead or alive.

I told you I was getting no information about Don's condition whatsoever, although the legal papers (of which you have copies) say that I am to have "unfettered visitation" with my husband and access to information regarding his medical condition.

I totally understand my husband's condition. I have accepted the fact that our marital relationship as we enjoyed it for so many years is no more. I also know that I cannot take care of Don at home. I know Lewy body dementia and its twists and turns because I lived intimately with it. I love my husband, and I am bound to him. But visiting in your facility has become a daily risk because of the gossip and tattling, lies, and distrust. If I am perceived as Don's enemy to be watched and "set up," then I do no one any good by seeing him.

Most wives get to be with their husbands during illness; most wives get to bury their husbands. But not me. Our marriage vows were broken, not by us; by his children, and those who have participated with them.

The only response to my letter was that the supervisor said she wished I had not mentioned her question regarding our finances. The staff did seem to take sides at this point, and they all did everything they could to accommodate me within their limitations.

Don's daughters were relentless in their effort to make my visits with Don as uncomfortable as possible. They stripped me of every right and privilege of being his wife. They seemed to be intent on overpowering me at every opportunity. A letter to my attorney from theirs read, "The parties previously agreed that Carol would be allowed to visit Don M-F from 11:00 am to 1:00 pm. My clients are also generally willing to allow her to visit on weekends, but request that it be during a scheduled period of time that is agreed upon before hand." I was incensed by the language. Was I supposed to be grateful because they were *"willing to allow"* me to visit my husband? Don was being treated like a prisoner, and I was being treated like a criminal, certainly not his wife of sixteen years.

Upon walking in one day, several pictures had been added to the ever-present family collage on the wall. There were two pictures of Don and his first wife together, probably taken in the 1970s. This was like a slap in my face! What were they thinking to exploit Don in such a way? He didn't even recognize who it was in the pictures, so it was not for his benefit that they were there, but obviously another message to me that they did not consider me Don's wife. I left them there and put a Post-it note on them, saying, "Nice touch, Kate." The pictures disappeared after Kate's next visit.

In a nursing home, visits do not normally last more than ten to twenty minutes. In that length of time, visitors can assess the condition of the patient and convince themselves that all is well. When Don's children came to visit, they came together, visiting with one another in Don's presence. All seemed well. I came to stay. I was with him every day for at least two hours, and most of that time, Don was in a deep sleep. While he slept, I visited with the other residents or caregivers, read, or just sat holding Don's hand as thoughts sped through my mind, or I studied Don's face and movements. I heard every conversation. I saw every stain on the floor. I noticed every time there was an inadequacy in his living conditions. And the inadequacies were many. This nursing home cost approximately $5,000 per month. For that $5,000, in this particular facility, there were no handicapped showers or toilets, there was no icemaker in the refrigerator, residents sat on plastic outdoor patio chairs in place of dining room chairs, the curtains were literally ragged, sometimes there was no soap in the bathrooms, and there were two flea infestations since Don arrived. For six residents with varying stages of dementia, there was only one caregiver. This is woefully inadequate. It is not humanly possible to take care of that many needy people with one caregiver. I insisted that for $5,000 per month, the residents should at least have ice in their tea, and soon a new refrigerator was brought in (I dubbed it the "Carol Pendergrass Memorial Refrigerator and Icemaker"). New dining room chairs were ordered. After I found live fleas in Don's bed, the house was treated for fleas.

Finding a New Normal

Most days, Don was pleasant and content in the home. Don was always a gentleman of the old sort: gracious, kind, polite, and patient, and best of all, he found value in every human being and showed respect for everyone. Those traits seemed magnified in his illness. He said little, but sometimes he would pound his imaginary gavel on the table, demand the attention of all, and give a long speech! His words seldom made sense, and his delusions were constant. He demanded that I come into his delusions with him. He would tell me he was beginning a new job and wanted to know how I was going to help him. A simple answer was not good enough. He would be ready to go to a meeting or on a trip and demanded that we leave together. He would want me to tell him the details of a delusional situation that I knew nothing about. He would become frustrated with me when I could not be present in his place of existence.

One Sunday morning, I was stealing time with Don. As we sat at the table with his housemates, Don's son Dale, who lived out of town, and his two children came into the house. They never spoke to me or acknowledged my presence. I slipped into Don's bedroom to wait. Don didn't seem to know who they were, but he was welcoming and polite, and then he sought me out in the bedroom while Dale and the children toured the facility with the caregiver. Dale made a comment to the caregiver that they just didn't know what I had done to Don—that he had been playing basketball just a few months ago, and now he was "like this." Don clung to me as they said their good-byes. When I asked him if he enjoyed their visit, he said he didn't know who they were.

Don never served in a war or the armed forces, and that seemed to be his one regret in life. He always thought it would have been a valuable life experience. So when he was making up his own reality, he was often at war, or preparing for flights he was piloting, or protecting his loved ones from the destruction of war.

He had constant hallucinations of snakes. He was not afraid of them; they were just always there. I asked him once what he thought of when he saw the snakes. He said, "Something that shouldn't be here. Something God doesn't want here." There were no walls to keep these creatures out. If he heard news on the television, he thought it was about him or his family. It was especially sad when he told me that one of the grandkids was killed in a car accident that day. He often had very grim, dark hallucinations. He believed the doctors were coming to do brain surgery on him; he was being beheaded; his hands or feet were being amputated; or he must wear an iron shoe that was being tightened. I suppose all of these delusions were based on a physical need or pain, but it made them no less horrific. Where he was, there was no sun to burn away the fog that obscured reality, so he had to live with the terrors in his mind, with no morning in which to wake.

To think about the long empty hours he had to fill with thoughts that haunted him with no relief or resolution was beyond my ability to endure. I quickly closed off those thoughts of what was going on in his mind in his solitude.

Don's children never seemed to accept the diagnosis of Lewy body. Back in May, in our home, I had asked Doug if he knew anything about LBD. I gave him a concise pamphlet on it, and he very animatedly tossed it aside without even looking at it. He was obviously giving me the message that he was not interested in that diagnosis. They didn't understand the nature of what Don was going through. Lewy body is a disease that runs in stages or phases. The only constants are the delusions and the hallucinations.

As time passed in the nursing home, he definitely knew that I was his wife and that he wanted me with him as a wife should be. Dementia does not take away the need for intimacy. Don wanted and needed to touch and be touched; to love and be loved. We lay together, as intimately as was possible, and he would press against me and whisper into my ear that he wanted to go home and make love with me.

In a light moment I said to him one day, "Do you still love me?" He answered, "Of course …. Inter-course!" and smiled broadly.

Sometimes, we spent the hours together drawing pictures on his legal pad. I am no artist, but my simple cat or dog seemed to entertain him and give him something to focus on. Don had been quite a good poet in his day, writing his feelings of love to me on cards and notes. One day I wrote, "I love you, your wife, Carol," on the pad, and he took the pen and wrote:

> "Carol, on a prescene of a rainy eve knight
> that penetrates you
> joyfully which continues
> a penetration of your special money
> *I Love You, Forever*"

Obviously, he had deep emotions that he wanted to express, but he no longer had the ability to find the words.

During the days of the civil suit, the children apparently talked to Don about what they were doing and explained it all in detail. He told me details of the lawsuit and warned me that they were seeking "the death penalty." He knew far too much about the suit to have made it up. They gave him all this information, and he had no way of interpreting it. He often thought he was in jail. He was greatly upset that this conflict was going on between the people he loved. He referred to "our side" and "the other side." I never knew on which side I fell. He seemed to always believe we were separated or divorced. He talked of the day when he and I could "reconcile" and be married again.

The day of our seventeenth anniversary came while Don was at the nursing home. I wanted to make it special for us and asked, a week in advance, for permission to take him out to dinner. The nursing home staff was doing their best to make this happen, but no word came from Kate. Finally, on the Saturday of our anniversary, the staff tried once again, and Kate simply said no. I kept thinking this would not bother me; I was expecting it. But when the word *no* came and we were refused the right to even celebrate our anniversary together, I broke. I didn't even mention my birthday in November. Being with him on holidays was impossible because the kids would take him to their homes for the day. In December, his seventieth birthday came. I knew I couldn't take him out, so I planned a party at the home and said I would bake his favorite cake. The administrator was there, and she told me I could not bake a cake and bring it in. They still were acting under the accusation of the kids that I might poison Don (and everyone else in the home, too, apparently). Again, I should have expected it, but when I was told I "could bring the ingredients and the staff would bake it" (come on; I could just as easily poison the ingredients! This is not about fear of poisoning—just meanness), I could not hold back the tears, and once I began, I could not stop. How much more could these children rob me of?

God Speaks to Me

Throughout the year, I prayed and believed that God would set the record straight. I believed that God would "show them," as we used to say when we were kids. I believed justice would come and God would rescue Don and me from the lies and abuse *because that is what I wanted*. But after months of escalating problems, I began to accept the fact that suffering is universal, and necessary; rarely does God rescue us. Still, I prayed earnestly for God to give me the strength I would need to get through this. Genesis 50:20 says, "What was meant for evil, God will turn for good." I clung to that scripture, praying that if I must go through this, that God would turn this hatred toward something good. That is God's way; to take sin and give us mercy; to take sorrow and give us joy in the morning; to take death and give us life everlasting. Although those scriptures are meaningful to us, until we are sustained by them, their meaning can seem vague.

We had a lovely home on a lake with a large yard, mature trees, and lots of space. I have a penchant for old, weathered cement garden pieces. Don had sighed many a time when I asked him to move another old fountain, statue, or urn into our yard. One piece was a three-tiered fountain so huge and heavy that I waited for Father's Day, when all six of our boys were at our house, to spring it on them. It took all six of them to set it up. It was in five pieces, each one weighing more than the last. In the summer, it was a lovely old fountain; in the winter, it held birdseed that the hungry birds and squirrels burrowed through the snow to feed on.

During the winter of Don's illness, it had collapsed somehow. The two smaller bowls had fallen on the lower, larger bowl and broken it in pieces. In the spring, the grass was coming up, but not under the huge broken bowl. I went outside to see what I could do with it, knowing it was too heavy for me to lift. I got a sledgehammer out of the garage and broke up the largest bowl into manageable pieces and loaded them in my little wagon. I studied what was left and thought if I could get the other two bowls up on the pedestal, it would still be a beautiful and useful piece, albeit not as large. The remaining largest bowl was over two feet across and made of solid concrete. I worked with it, rolling it, wedging it, jacking it up, using all the tricks I could think of, but I could not get it up on the twelve-inch-high pedestal. Of course, I tried lifting it, but that was impossible.

I felt I would have to wait for help, when that voice I know said to go inside, get something to drink, come back, and try again, and I would have the strength. I had been praying for the strength to go on and not be defined by what was happening to me. I constantly prayed for strength to get through the lawsuits, Don's illness, and our financial difficulties, and prayed to be a loving wife, mother, and grandmother. I obeyed the voice in my soul. After a slow drink of tea, I went back outside, set my feet apart on each side of the huge concrete bowl, reached down, and put my hands on it, and I lifted it, turned with it, and set it on the pedestal! No one could have been more surprised than me. I had not struggled. My back did not hurt. How did that just happen? I sat down and simply laughed! God had just showed me that if He could give me the strength to do the impossible, He would give me all the strength I would ever need to get through this situation.

The reality of Don's being in a nursing home, never to return to our home, was setting in. In July, I awoke at midnight. I had been sleeping on Don's side of the bed, and from there, I awoke and looked straight down the hallway. It was completely dark, and I had never felt so alone. In that twilight moment between wake and sleep,

I began to despair. As I looked into the black hallway, the voice in my soul that I know to be God's said, *"Everything is as it should be."* I knew God had spoken to me and let me know He was aware of all that was going on. He was in charge, and though we were apart, *Don was where he needed to be and I was where I should be.* I closed my eyes in peace and slept. Those words have rung in my soul every single day. I always thought that if God really spoke to us we would not, could not, ever forget what He said. And those words are just as real today as they were that dark night.

These experiences, Rebecca's prayer, and many other blessings that God sent my way, including the outpouring of prayers and the love from others, will be with me forever. People whom I had never met before, who crossed my path during this time, would stop me to say they would pray for me. I knew there was a divine purpose in their presence. I sat across from a stranger in a nail salon and she looked at me and said, "I am going to mass to pray for you." That was the extent of our conversation, and I have never seen her again. I have come to look for God in everything, for I believe He is there. I believe God is aware of us, and our circumstances. And I believe God desires to intervene in our lives. I have that "perfect peace" the Bible tells us about, and I know it comes from God.

No Laws, No Justice

On June 25, for the first time in my life, I was called to jury duty. I almost laughed at the timing. Sitting in judgment of another person was the last place I wanted to be when my own lawsuits were pending … three of them. But perhaps there was a reason that I should go, observe and learn about the system I would soon face myself. It was my intention to disqualify myself at the first opportunity and get out of there.

I was scheduled to sit on a civil case. The jury pool was questioned. All I could think was that I would soon be sitting in that same defendant's chair, and I was frightened. During the first round of questioning, I told the judge I could not stand in judgment of another. That didn't get me dismissed. On the second day of the process, he asked if there was anyone in the pool who could not accept the testimony of a police officer as truth. Now this was something I could honestly answer! I raised my hand and said that due to two recent situations, where I felt unjustly dealt with, I was not exactly a believer in the credibility of the police force. I was dismissed.

What I did learn from being in the courtroom was that I did not want to sit in that defendant's chair. The longer I looked at it, the more it looked like an electric chair. The courtroom is a land I do not know or understand; where tricks are played and the craftiest attorney wins. I was no longer sure truth or justice had anything to do with it, and I really began to pray for a way to avoid that chair.

Through our attorneys, we continued to work on a settlement. From the start, I knew I could not successfully fight the guardianship/conservatorship that Kate and Carla had taken. Nor did I particularly want to. Ideally, I would have wanted the girls to have medical power of attorney for Don, and I would have the right to control our own assets and money, but I so wanted these people out of my life that I was ready to let them have the power they wanted. (Was this what it was about? A power struggle?) Every day, I lived in fear that they would come into our house and take what they wanted. I feared that they would freeze my bank accounts so that I could not even pay my bills. I feared that I had not even imagined yet what they were capable of taking from me. Every time a car drove up, I was afraid that I would be served with some new petition or charge. I was tired of living in fear of these people. From the beginning, I had outlined a plan whereby I would grant Kate and Carla permanent guardianship and conservatorship of Don. I would sign over all of our joint assets to his conservancy account and retain only what was mine personally. When we married, Don had his own townhouse, to which I never laid claim (although it was titled in joint tenancy). They had already taken over his Social Security income and a small oil and gas royalty income. I just wanted them to take the assets and assume his debts on them. This meant I would sign over the Quarry, and they could deal with Frank and leave me out of that conflict.

Our attempts at settlement, even the grueling meeting that I'd had with their attorneys to present documentation of our financial position, did not satisfy Don's children. On the day that we were expecting to receive a settlement plan, we were notified that Don's children had fired their law firm and hired another. Again I was dumbfounded. I assumed that when the lawyers who had questioned me reported that there was no case and that I was not guilty of the accusations, they were fired. My attorney was told that the lawyer who was fired spent four hours with Kate and Carla and could not persuade them that settling was in their interest. He was told the firm had not been "aggressive enough," and Don's kids wanted "a pound of flesh." The only way this made any sense to the two attorneys was if Don's children had come to believe their own lie, that I deliberately tried to kill Don. The attorney said, "I don't think you can spend ten minutes with her and believe she deliberately tried to injure Don."

So we were back at the beginning, thousands of dollars spent on attorneys, and absolutely no ground gained. I was ordered to appear for a formal deposition, which was to take place on September 4. In the meantime, we prepared for a trial. I knew I had done nothing wrong. We filed with the court the formal legal rebuttal to the lawsuit, which is called the "Answer." We presented *thirty-seven points of rebuttal*, all of which could be proven. I turned over my journal, which is approximately a four-inch-thick notebook, containing a daily log of everything that had happened since Don began to lose his cognitive abilities. It also contained every e-mail or letter or document that passed between Don's children and me. That journal became very valuable to me, as many entries or e-mails showed the accusations against me to be false or intentional lies. The attorneys subpoenaed all doctor's records, hospital records, hospice records, care home records … anything that could be used in the court case, for or against me, as part of the discovery. I was very confident and wanted to go to trial. I knew we could refute the charges and win this suit, and I was looking forward to the opportunity to finally be able to be heard.

At the pretrial hearing, which is a private meeting between the judge and the attorneys, the judge (who had signed the original ex parte order and who would be hearing the case) told my attorney that he would be "pissed" if this came before him. Besides, the court had so little respect for my rights that the judge had allotted only a few hours for our case, should it go to court, so that we could not even begin to present our case. The judge ordered the attorneys to settle this and not bring it to trial.

This news devastated me. I was not going to be able to be heard. I was refused my right to a trial. That left me with no alternative but to give in and settle with them, whatever that would be. No matter what the truth was or who was telling it, I would lose because accusations had been made, and I would not have the opportunity to be heard.

My attorneys told me that if I defied the judge's admonition and pursued the case to court, it would take possibly years to get a decision and cost as much as $35,000 more in legal fees before it was finished. The attorneys obviously did not want to prolong my case. Under this kind of lawsuit, compensation for attorney's fees would not be awarded, so no matter the outcome, I would be responsible for my own fees. And if I lost, it would obviously be financially devastating to me. James knew all of this going in. Doug knew this going in. I did not. I still believed in justice and the law and the upholding of marriage vows. I was wrong on all three counts. There would be no justice for me.

Waiting on the Train

July 17, 2007

I remember when I was impatient. Impatient to grow up; to fall in love and begin my "real" life; impatient for the days and months to pass me on to new adventures. Now the days, months, years have gained so much momentum that I rarely know the date. And patience is much more than just waiting to come ... or go. It is waiting on things to change, and fall into place, and to be content, even happy in the waiting. For six months now I've been waiting, learning to be patient, as I watch the battle that is now my life. I'm waiting on the train that comes close, runs over my toes, and speeds up again to make another round. Patience has been not being able to go away because I can't risk missing the train, but not knowing when it might come and run over me again. (from my journal)

Don started a phase of sleeping all the time. One of the hallmarks of Lewy body is that there are distinct phases that come and go. When Don was home, I could sense a new phase coming and tell when he was going to start a new pattern, and then it would pass into something else after a week or so. Now Don could not be awakened out of his deep sleep, and if he awoke, he would fall asleep in midsentence.

His delusions and hallucinations continued. He saw children, animals, boats, airplanes, and always snakes. He would look at a picture on the wall and see something completely different. I began to wonder if he could see at all. I wondered about what he saw when I walked in. I began to experiment and to observe him closely. I concluded that he still had prosopagnosia, or "face blindness," and did not recognize one person from another until they spoke to him. Prosopagnosia is a failure to *recognize*, not because they have forgotten people or because their eyes are not working but because the brain is not able to put together information properly. It is not a problem of memory. Every day I would come in, saying the same words: "Hi, honey." I don't believe he knew my face, but he recognized my words and then knew our relationship. His memories of emotion were still working. If I showed him a picture of the two of us, he did not know me, and he did not know himself, either. When he had visitors, he would act as though he knew who they were, although he did not. He was pleasant and polite and warm to everyone, so no one guessed.

Don wanted more than anything to go outside the home. He was childlike in his attempts to get out of the house. His insistence that I take him out was relentless. He would become upset, weepy, and desperate, and he accused me, saying, "This sounds like a divorce," he suspected that there was someone else, that I was lying, that I just didn't want to be with him anymore. These accusations crushed me, especially under the circumstances where I was forbidden to take him out without reason. Many times I left the home weeping out of frustration because Don was angry with me and was accusing me of infidelity.

Much of the time at the home, I felt I was trying to fit where I didn't belong. I was not sure who I was to Don—wife, caregiver, just another visitor. Some days I felt I was pressing an issue that no longer existed. One day Don said to me, "What is our relationship?" When I said I was his wife, he looked confused and said, "You can't just leave one in the dust and get a new one." I began to cry inside. He closed his eyes and retreated deep inside himself. I thought he was asleep. Then without opening his eyes he said, "I want to be with you forever."

I was around the nursing home enough to sense things and to have conversations with the caregivers. We became friends. I would ask a lot of questions about Don's behavior in the home. Professional caretakers keep the negative behavior from the families of their charges. Unless there is a medical problem, they consider this behavior their problem, which they are paid to handle. So Don's children were never told that he became combative and violent over a shower or hygiene issues. They never knew that he refused to allow the caregivers to change him or give him medications. They never knew that he ransacked his room during the night and refused to get into his bed and physically fought with the caregivers when they tried to help him. I had lived with this behavior, so I could usually tell when he was in those phases. When I was with Don, he became calm, and the caregivers would give a sigh of relief. Many times I showered him or shaved him, or accompanied him to the bathroom when he refused to go with the staff. When I became discouraged about my visits, the staff would tell me that I was Don's stability, his calming spirit; that when I wasn't there, it was like something was missing for him. And I would be encouraged to keep trying to fit.

There were those wonderful moments of clarity that I lived for. I sat beside him one day as he slept. He opened his eyes and looked at me, and I softly said, "I love you." He said, "I'm not the person you loved." He said after all he'd been through, he'd changed and was a different person. I told him I still loved him and told him what mattered was that he still loved me. He put his arm around me and held me against his chest and said, "More now than I ever have."

The light bulb flickered.

Don and I sat around the table with the other residents; we were the only couple. Over and over the housemates asked the same questions (because they could not remember from a moment ago when they last asked): "Where did you meet that old frog? How long have you been together?" In hopes of stirring Don's memory, I would tell stories of things we did together. Sometimes he seemed to remember; sometimes he asked me not to tell those lies. Once we were discussing Don's gentle spirit with the staff, and I said, "Even if I wanted to fight, Don would not fight!" Don sat quietly, and with his half-smile I knew so well, he simply replied, "I'm a coward."

Don continued to talk to me about the lawsuit. He told me once, "Give the kids what they want so we can settle this!" I asked, "Have your kids been talking to you about this?" He told me yes, that he knew all about it. He knew they had sued me. He often asked me if I had received "the papers" or if I had "given them the money." The caregivers told me that during one conversation, lawyers were mentioned. They commented to Don that he had lawyers in the family, and he said, "Yes, too damn many!"

One day when I sat down with Don, I was stunned to see amidst the eternal collage a picture of Frank sitting with Don on the couch in the nursing home. Now the kids were bringing Frank, the adversary, to visit with Don. How could this be right, when I was fighting a lawsuit with him, and his only claim to our property was that Don told him something in private? There was no more sense in this than in anything else that had happened. I challenged the right of the conservator of Don's estate to fraternize with Frank during this lawsuit, but as always, it fell on deaf ears.

During the days at the care home, the caretakers and I became friends and shared a lot of time together. I told them I was going to have to write a book about this experience, and we began to playfully cast who would play our roles in the movie. Queen Latifah would play the caretaker, Harrison Ford would be Don, and Sally Field would play me. Apparently our friendship wasn't as close as I thought it was, and the caretaker told Frank about our jesting conversation. In one of several long, vile letters Frank later wrote to me, he said, "Sorry to tell you, that book and movie has already been written and the movie made. The name of the movie was *Misery* [Stephen King's thriller about torture and imprisonment] and your role was played by Kathy Bates." I gasped in disbelief and threw the letter down as if it had come from hell itself; I know now who is really demented.

For a few months, I was told that Frank visited Don every other week. During this time, in a quiet moment, Don told me he thought

Frank was going to show up and cause some trouble. He warned me to stay away from him. I was told Frank ceased to visit after those first months.

In October, Don began to tell me he thought he was being poisoned.

"It Is What It Is"

I wanted to be exonerated. I wanted to be avenged. I wanted to be heard and all the accusations proven to be lies. I wanted the judge, like Judge Judy, to put Don's children in their place and shame them for what they had done! I wanted to be made whole. My attorney was quick to tell me that was not what was going to happen in this case. I knew I had done nothing to harm my husband or any of the other things I'd been accused of, so why wouldn't I be found faultless and exonerated? It was very important to me that it be made known to the powers-that-be that I was not guilty and all the charges were shamefully bogus. Constantly, my thinking was to *change the situation* to reflect my innocence. The whole situation was repugnant to me, and instinctively I argued every point. At the time, I couldn't understand what my attorney was trying to tell me, but he finally said, "Carol, it is what it is." I finally realized with those words that I had to start where we were—and accept the reality of the situation and quit trying to make it something that I wanted it to be. This was a mean, unfounded lawsuit brought about by people who wanted to hurt me. It was not about truth or justice; but about destroying me. That was difficult to accept. We had been a family. But that is what it was.

I began to look at everything in the light of those words. My life was just what it was. Don's illness was what it was. Having to settle with these people was what it was. I had to accept things as they were and go from there.

I suppose many people do not have lifelong friends. I have been blessed to have several friends since my childhood, who have only grown closer through the years. My dearest friend, Pamela Landis, and I have been best friends since the first day of eighth grade in 1960. In our adult years, we moved to different states, but we never moved away from each other emotionally. We have shared the joys of our lives and the disappointments, the births of our sons (on the same day), and everything in between. Before Don and I were married, Pam and I tried to spend a week together each year. She had been my confidant through my life, and throughout this year she had kept me out of the therapist's office. I could always say to Pam what I could not say to anyone else (sometimes even to myself). It was time for me to go to her. Pam and I had long talked of our granddaughters, who were almost the same age, hoping that the girls could meet and maybe find in each other a little of what she and I had shared throughout our lives. In August, my granddaughter, Erin, and I boarded a plane for San Diego. I kissed Don good-bye for two weeks and escaped with Erin to sandy beaches and Disneyland.

As I tried to put my everyday world behind me, my attorney was preparing for my deposition, which was to take place as soon as I returned. I did not want to think about any of that, but the web was being spun even while I was gone.

On September 3, my deposition took place. How intimidating to be in a room full of attorneys, the focus of all eyes and all questions. Doug, an attorney himself, was present, along with his new attorney (who replaced the one they had fired), Don's court-appointed attorney, my attorney, a court stenographer, and me. I was not afraid; more like angry. I was incensed that I had to answer personal questions that were no one else's business. We started midmorning and left the law office about seven that evening. It was very intense. I was asked the questions I knew would be asked about my intentions and actions regarding Don and his illness. Doug's attorney asked me, if it had been up to me to take care of Don, what arrangements would I have made and how would I have done it? I was so glad to have an opportunity to answer that question! My answer was "Thank you for asking me that. *You are the first one to even ask me.*" The fact that Don's children had assumed that I would or would not do certain things, but never brought it up or asked, was one of the most insane things about this case.

I was asked if Don and I slept in the same bed, and when we stopped. I was asked about the names I have gone by (as though they would find me on a wanted poster). I was asked questions about my son's personal life. I was asked about the purchase of my car, with the accusation that I had taken Don's money and bought an expensive new car and deprived him of what was his! I was asked about my trip to California. "Did you go alone?" the attorney asked, as though they had caught me with another man. Every move I made was suspect. I was asked about visiting Don. I said I saw him every day unless it was impossible for me to be there. The attorney said, "What would make it impossible?" I said, "Well, I'm not there today!" and hoped I made my point. Many questions were personal and unrelated to the situation, and I would refuse to answer. But in a deposition, that is not an option. I was directed by my attorney to answer.

That bothersome curse to find humor in everything kept taunting me as I thought how little and perfect the attorney's teeth were; I began to count them. I didn't want to answer his questions. I wanted to ask him if he had worn braces and how much they had cost.

We took a few breaks, and I accompanied my attorney outside when he smoked. I said, "Give me one of those," although I'd never had a cigarette in my mouth before. I thought now would be an excellent time to start. I didn't drink either, but if we had been near a bar, I could have downed a few!

Back in the deposition, many of the questions were misquotes that I was asked to explain. I would refer to my journal, find the page, and read what the actual conversation had been, or read the e-mail showing the truth of the situation. I had a feeling that the attorneys all thought my corpulent journal was silly, but Don had always told me to "write it down," and that in a court of law, it would be the written word that would prevail. Having the details of every day to refer to made me feel secure and saved me from false accusations several times.

I was asked whether I thought Don should be in a nursing home. I adamantly agreed that he should, but said I wasn't crazy about the one he was presently in. Asked why I felt that way, I began to list the things I had seen in the home—no ice, plastic chairs, not enough supervision, and inadequate bathroom facilities. When I got to the fleas, my attorney stopped me and said, in exasperation, "Other than that, Mrs. Lincoln, did you enjoy the play?" I began to laugh hysterically at that, but he and I seemed to be the only ones who "got" it.

The long day went on; the questions seemed silly. The whole experience seemed mad and contrived and senseless. Absolutely no new information was gained; it just seemed an exercise in intimidation. It wasn't one of those things where you can judge who might have won. I had no idea what conclusions were drawn or even what it was all about, unless it was purely for intimidation.

During the days and weeks after the deposition, we tried to work out an acceptable settlement. E-mails were going back and forth rapidly, but as soon as we would come to an agreement, we would hear nothing for a week or more. I was always afraid that the new law firm had been fired and we would have to start over again. Then, when we did hear back, the children would decide to change it all, and come up with some new, bizarre thing they wanted, which was always unacceptable to our side. One thing that came out of nowhere was that they wanted me to agree to set up a scholarship in Don's name. This scholarship would be funded by a portion of the cash remaining in the conservancy upon Don's death. Because of the implications of that action to me, it was summarily rejected. As the negotiations flew back and forth, we received an e-mail from Doug's attorney. He had intended to "cut and paste" some text in the interest of time, but he inadvertently sent Doug's entire e-mail to us.

For me, this letter was the turning point in everything that had happened so far and everything that would happen in the future. Doug's letter to his attorney outlining his intentions was mean-spirited and arrogant. I believe he was confident that they would force me to settle under their terms. He stated that they would press me hard "on the risk the civil action presents" in order to "motivate" me to settle. He outlined how they would use the scholarship as a bargaining tool—saying they would concede, in increments, the amount pledged to the scholarship in relation to the amount of time I would give up being with my husband (forcing me to buy my time with him). His argument was that they were "on high moral ground," because they said Don had a "soft spot" for scholarships. Doug said he believed I had "some ability to feel shame," so forcing me to bid against a scholarship in Don's name with each exchange of offers, would "take a psychological toll" on me.

He stated they would hold as fact, and their testimony in court would be:

- That I tied Don up, which Doug says is a crime
- That I did not give Don his medication as prescribed
- That I said his kids should be financially responsible for Don's care
- That I actively discouraged the children from giving Don food and water when they visited him in our home
- That a jury would see my "motive" because I transferred "jointly held assets" into my trust while being unwilling to place Don in appropriate care
- And, "the general theme" was that I had the "opportunity to take care of him properly but didn't"

The last point of Doug's letter said they would drive me into bankruptcy, and that my home, other assets, and my future income would "be at risk" if I did not settle. He also said, "If we get a judgment, <u>we will dog her for the rest of her life</u> in order to execute on assets and garnish wages."

Finally, he said they were "<u>determined and financially able to continue the civil action</u>" against me, if I did not settle under their terms.

I was appalled. I felt defeated.

I didn't think I could be hurt by their words any more, but this letter cut me to the bone. Somewhere in my heart, I guess I hoped they didn't really hate me, but this left no doubt. I realized that I didn't have a chance in hell to ever win anything against these people, who were liars and manipulators. They proved that it was "about the money," at least about keeping my own money from me, when they demanded half of the remaining conservancy be given to a scholarship program. What was in the conservancy was all of our assets; our life savings; all I would ever have; our retirement. During our marriage, Don never gave to any scholarship program, not even to his own alma mater. If Don had a "soft spot" for any charity, it was Special Olympics, which they did not seem to know. Don's children had so many misconceptions about their father that I often wondered who they were talking about. The arrogance of the children to think they would know a man better than his wife. Who knows what a man and his wife share in the darkness of the early morning hours? Certainly not these children. The plans we made together; our hopes and dreams for each other; the intimate and sometimes painful discussions of our future years in life and death; these children knew nothing of this relationship. In this letter they were hoping to drive me into bankruptcy. How did this honor their father?

Now, with this letter, at least I knew who these people really were. I knew now that I had lost the case and my only hope was to secure a reasonably acceptable settlement.

PART THREE

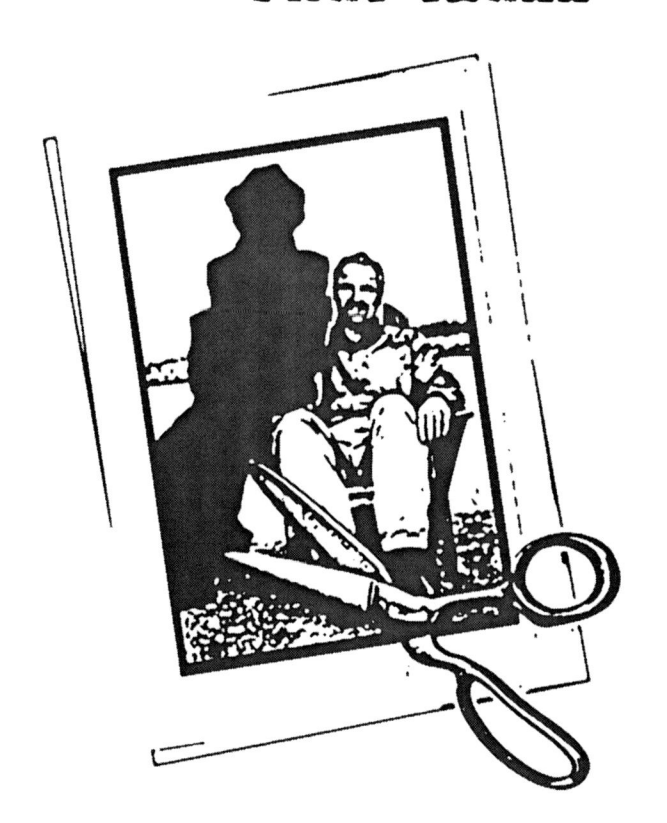

Discovery

In the weeks after seeing Doug's e-mail, I lost hope. I didn't even know if I could come out of this with enough to live on. I was worried they would find a way to take my house or maybe, just for the heck of it, refuse to settle with me at all just to keep my life in turmoil, as Doug had suggested. Their hatred seemed to have no limits. What was it that drove their hatred? It had been a very long time since I'd had self-doubt. Don gave me confidence. Because he believed in me, I believed in myself. And because I knew I'd done no wrong, my confidence had not waned, up to now. But Doug's e-mail was vile. I guess I could accept that they wanted what they wanted, but I never thought they could be so full of hate. From the beginning, why hadn't they just asked for what they wanted? What was I missing? What was I not seeing clearly? Could I be this bad person Don's children believed me to be? In my despair, my family and friends became even stronger for me. Friends from Kansas City often came just to make sure I was all right. Everyone I knew stayed close by me. My son, Rob, was always there with strong support, encouragement, and love. In one of my lowest moments, he said to me, "Mom, they had to call four policemen to accompany them. You come with an army of people who truly love you." I remember those words often and find peace and comfort in them.

Doug was right about one thing: I did have the ability to feel shame. I was ashamed of these people I had once regarded as my children. Although I would always be proud to be Don's wife, I was now ashamed of having the same name as his children.

The latter part of Doug's e-mail was full of lies. He referred to a note in which he said I admitted that I "tied Dad up." That note was from a journal entry about a violent evening when Don was in a terrible psychosis. He had literally ransacked our kitchen, had torn his clothes off, and was totally out of control of his bodily functions. The kitchen looked like a cow barn in winter. He was in a rage his children could not imagine. I could not get control of the situation. I opened a pill bottle with my teeth and managed to grab a Haldol tablet, which the doctor had given me in the event of such a situation, but Don hit me and the tablet flew out of my hand and disappeared. My thoughts were racing, and I knew I had to have help, but who could help me? Who could come into this situation and understand it? This scene was humiliating and sickening. I had been told in such a situation to call the police or fire department, but I couldn't get to the phone. Don backed up against the refrigerator, and in my desperation, I prayed aloud for him to "be still." He stopped cold, and while I held him with one hand, I pulled his wheelchair up with the other. He sank into the chair, and I tied him into it with the terry cloth belt from my robe. Doug knew full well that the Kansas law to which he referred is for professional facilities and not for home care of a spouse. The rest of that paragraph of Doug's e-mail was what I could expect to occur on the witness stand: half-truths and misrepresentations of the facts.

Doug used an admission he said I made on May 5, 2007, that I "did not give medications as prescribed." This came from a note on the hospital report when Don was admitted with the bowel impaction. I told the hospital personnel that he had not taken his medications regularly for about a week because during his psychosis, he would violently refuse to take them or he would not swallow them and would spit them across the room. Of course this resulted in him not getting his medications regularly, and I thought it was important that the doctors know that. It is a blatant lie that I "actively discouraged" them from giving Don food or water. Common sense defies such a statement! Kate challenged me once that Don did not have fresh water, which was not true, and she started to argue with me when Doug chided her to stop. Kate was invited to (and did) refill his water. I told them they were welcome to the refrigerator where there was pudding, soups, Jell-O, or anything they wanted. I doubt if they understood he was on a soft food diet. Sherry had testified that I provided the best food within his diet and that we fed him as much as he was able to eat. Where this absurd accusation came from was beyond me. But absurdity seemed to be the order of the day for Doug and his siblings.

Doug wrote that in a meeting I said Don's kids should be financially responsible for his care. What I said was that if they were so concerned that I would not be able to take care of Don with our own money, and they *wanted control*, maybe they would like to start a trust for their dad and contribute to his care. I actually thought it was a little humorous. I was enraged that they would try to step in and demand control of our finances, assuming that I would not take care of him! What I said to Doug was that when Doug gave me his financials to prove to me that he was able to take care of his children properly, then I would show him ours. I simply could not have said anything that would have *not* been construed as abusive behavior to their father. Like Alice in the court of the Queen of Hearts, truth had no place here, and every fact was twisted and changed to their advantage. The verdict was already in, and it was "Off with her head" no matter what I did.

Doug's e-mail was so full of lies, hatred, and evil that I was scared to death what a trial might look like. Doug *never* knew that we received his wayward e-mail.

During the long months of the settlement negotiations, still preparing for further depositions that were being scheduled, and still under the threat of the accusations of trying to kill my husband, the subpoenaed records from the various institutions, doctors, and EMS were beginning to accumulate. Again, being attorneys, both James and Doug already had these records and had taken from the documents what they chose to use against me. I was most anxious to see what they had already seen that would give any substantiation to their claims. Finally, the subpoenaed records were in my hands. This would turn out to be the most difficult to swallow of all that had been offered up to me, and it is now the most difficult to relate.

These records are part of what is called "Discovery." This process involves seeing what information each side has that they will use to prove or disprove the case in a trial. We would be discovering exactly what took place during the last year. I was absolutely confident that the facts were going to fall into place, and I would finally be exonerated.

But seeing the "facts" in black and white do not give "cause." I read every note from every doctor and every report that was made regarding Don's treatment. At last I hoped I would find out what happened on that fateful Sunday afternoon in February.

A report from February 26, 2007, described Don's first visit with Dr. R, his psychologist, after being taken from our home. It is a lengthy, detailed report, but very telling. Dr. R reported that on this visit, Don *"appeared to have a body odor, unkempt hair, disheveled dress and appearance, which was a change from previous sessions. When asked what was going on, [Don] stated that he really did not know."* The psychologist's report said that Don's daughters had told him that on February 11, Don had called Carla and told her he felt unsafe. He said "the cleaning lady" had frightened him, and Carla explained that "Carol is the cleaning lady." Another doctor, in another report, said Don *"has difficulty in determining dreams from reality and vacillates in and out of reality during therapy today. He has an increasingly distorted perception of reality. When asked about his marriage, he said he thought he had been married three times; twice legally and once illegally. Family [children] is fearing for his safety and would like him hospitalized."* Obviously his children were experiencing the same thing I had gone through with Don, but they were still anxious to blame me. One quick call to me saying simply, "Dad called and said he is afraid. What is going on there?" and this whole terrible situation could have been avoided.

But I now believe they had been setting up, planning on, and waiting for that call.

The girls had reported that while he was at Kate's, he was hallucinating, was having delusions, and was increasingly paranoid; they were even afraid he might harm himself. These were the things I had been trying to tell them for weeks (except I never saw any indication of self-injurious behavior). And yet they chose to believe his delusions at home on that one Sunday afternoon.

The reports then escalated to Don being poisoned by his wife. Don *"described overhearing some women at work talking about that he was being poisoned,"* wrote one doctor. This is what he had also told me in a telephone conversation, that he had heard someone else say he was being poisoned, not that he believed he was being poisoned. A few days later, another doctor wrote, *"The daughter reports paranoid behavior and poisoning by his wife."* This statement came two weeks after they had taken him from me.

I learned what happened when Don said he ran away from a nursing home. Kate and Carla had taken him to a hospital behavioral unit (psych ward). *"Three weeks ago the patient was with his second wife and called the daughter to come get him because he was feeling unsafe. He has been staying with one of the daughters since then and was very confused when trying to give a history about why he is in the hospital today. He is not able to say he was at this daughter's house and is very circumstantial about his current condition. His* ex-wife *went to the daughter's house* demanding *to see the patient but the police were called and she was not allowed to see him."* I could do nothing but sit in disbelief when I read this. How could I demand to see Don when no one came to the door? And I was now Don's "ex-wife"? Their intentions became unquestionable. Every other document represented us as being "separated."

Don was admitted to the ward and endured tests for two days. Apparently Kate and Carla got the same bad feeling as I had from that place, and the documents said they decided Don wasn't *"that bad after all,"* and they took him out against medical advice, as I had. Much of their criticism of my actions was based on my allowing him to go AMA, when in fact they had done the same thing.

Another hospital document said *"history of physical, SEXUAL, emotional abuse"* was reported by daughters: "SEXUAL" was in capital letters. Exactly how do you sexually abuse a seventy-year-old man with dementia? If this had not been such an astonishing charge, it would have been funny. Time and again, the physician's reports repeated that the daughters had put it in the records that Don had been poisoned and abused. In at least one report, he was tested for poisoning but no trace was found, and yet the girls persisted in reporting poisoning to other doctors.

I was sickened with every report that showed the girls had given false information to the doctors. I was accused of causing his ailments from the bowel impaction to acute renal (kidney) failure. I did not know he was ever diagnosed with acute renal failure. When I saw that on the reports, I was shocked until I saw that it was actually "pre-renal," which means inadequate blood circulation to the kidneys caused by heart disease. Of course, the girls knew this but chose to pursue language that could be used against me.

One thing I was very anxious to see was the report from the EMS regarding Don's condition on May 16. It was unremarkable except that it showed that Don's blood pressure began dropping when they began to remove him; he was not in that condition, as the girls had said, in our home. The report actually showed that the action taken on the morning of May 16 was what caused the drop in blood pressure.

The documents confirmed that SRS and hospice were told of the ex parte order two days before I was. When the hospice nurse came the night before, she knew what was going to happen. The social worker and chaplain knew. Why did no one think that I should be told? I tried to figure out what they were thinking to let this cruelty happen as a total shock.

The hospice report made by the social worker on Tuesday, May 15, the day before they took him, read, *"Patient's daughter [Kate] reported that she and siblings are planning to move patient to [care home]. Kate reported that she has been granted guardianship."* There is a lengthy description of conversations with the care home, Kate, and Carla, whereby they wanted to trick me into moving Don by taking him to the in-patient hospice unit in the hospital and then transferring him to the nursing home. Hospice wrote, *"I informed them that we would not participate … as this would involve deception. I provided education on appropriate use of in-patient placement and informed [Kate] that the current situation was not an appropriate use."* Did hospice owe me nothing? No loyalty? The decency of just letting me know?

I found that SRS was supposedly still "investigating" me. The last I had heard from them was that they were actively pursuing Don's children for taking our money. The caregivers at the nursing home had said that when the SRS finished their investigation of me, "it would be over," but I believed they were misinformed. Now I found that the girls were still insisting on an investigation, and from the hospital records, I found that SRS was following Don's treatment. This was difficult to figure out. I finally came to the belief that SRS just didn't have the backbone to stand up against this family and played along with them at my (and the taxpayers') expense.

On May 16, Don was taken from our home to St. Francis Hospital, where he went through the same procedure he had gone through a week before. There was nothing new in any of the reports. He was there for two weeks and then transferred to Newton Hospital. During the deposition, the attorney asked me, "Do you admit that Don did improve after he was taken from your home?" I said it was apparent he had, then added, "but that is not to say that he would not have improved under my care." He had only been out of the hospital three days and had already begun to show improvement. The assumption that the girls were trying to make was had they not taken him from our home and to the hospital on May 16, he would have died due directly to my care.

Enough

I was tired of this whole thing. I was weary from being afraid all the time. I wanted out of this family. I wanted whatever it would take to have peace. I needed to go to sleep at night without these accusations hanging over my head and the surreal dreams they brought. My other life went on. I was a mother and a grandmother; I was a sister and a friend; I was depended upon to do my work and maintain the finances of others. I had a home to keep and bills to pay. I needed to feel secure enough to begin to fill the emptiness that the ravenous storm had left. I'd been afraid and grieving long enough. I wanted my life back!

On November 1, 2007, we finally reached a settlement. Basically, I agreed to give them all of our jointly owned assets, pay them a cash amount, pay half of Don's court-appointed attorney's fees, and let them keep all money they had taken from us and, of course, all of Don's personal real properties. I dropped any opposition to the guardianship and conservancy orders. My two personal real estate properties, my car, and the possessions in our home were mine. In exchange, all charges were dropped with prejudice (which means they can never be brought up again). They also *allowed* me to keep my personal bank accounts! In the event Don died before they used up all of the funds in the conservancy account, I will get 75 percent of the remainder, and Don's children will get the other 25 percent. I will be allowed to keep the insurance policies we had in place. I could live with this settlement. After all the shameful activities to get to this point, I felt very fortunate to have fared so well. At least I would be free of these children.

In January 2008, after the settlement agreement, Doug called from Texas and cheerily said he was coming to town and wanted to meet with me, take possession of Don's vehicle, and get some of Don's guns (which we had agreed upon in the settlement), and then we could share information and "talk." Now that they had won the game they were playing, they seemed to expect to return to our former relationship and have a freakin' party! I said, "That isn't going to happen. I'm not going to talk to any of you. If you want something from me, contact my attorney." Doug expressed surprise and shock that I would take such an attitude. I said simply, "You went too far," and hung up. My attorney met Doug at my home and turned over the keys to the truck and the guns to him. Doug, however, said that there were other guns, so I said if he didn't believe me, he could go through my closets, never dreaming he would. He did! Finding no guns, he asked about a handgun he said he remembered Don having. Don's revolver had never been brought up before and was never in our agreement. I always felt threatened by Frank, so having the gun gave me a sense of protection. However, Doug actually took the gun out of my bureau drawer and took it with him. Apparently even my attorney was intimidated by Doug; I felt he should not have allowed Doug to go through my closets or to take the handgun. The audacity of these people was beyond belief. The word *bully* kept coming to my mind. My reward is that they will never enter my home again.

Visitation

Part of our settlement agreement was that Don's court-appointed attorney would study our situation and draw up a "visitation plan" for me. I hoped that the plan would show me the respect of being Don's wife and drop the stupid limitations that had been applied to me. We waited four months for the plan. During those four months, Don was in rapid decline. Kate and Carla began to seek new doctors for aggressive treatment. In January 2008, Kate made an appointment to start Don on physical therapy. The Parkinson's symptoms were getting worse, and his legs had become almost useless. I highly objected to physical therapy because he had twice become violent after such treatment. Also, the girls did not seem to realize that it was not his legs that wouldn't work, but his mind. I knew if he went to physical therapy, he would become aggressive and probably end back up in the psych ward.

And that is exactly what happened. I arrived at the care home one morning and was told Don was not there; he was in the behavioral unit of the hospital (psych ward). Back in the Cuckoo's Nest. The supervisor of the home was upset that he was taken there, but Kate was making the decisions. When he was admitted (to the same place from which he had left AMA twice), they used restraints. I was told Kate forbade that, so he was put on a mattress on the floor. I could not bear to think of him being there, and what it was doing to him. He was there for ten days.

I was not allowed to see him or to inquire about him in the hospital. I told my attorney about this turn of events, and he appealed to the attorney drawing up the visitation plan. She still had not presented it to the court, but she called Kate personally and told her she was not to keep me from seeing Don. Kate said it was an "oversight" that I was not put on the visitation list. Oops! A code was required to even call about Don, and the attorney acquired the code for me. I was tired of asking how a wife of seventeen years was an "oversight."

I no longer asked, "How can I bear this?" I know. I just will. What else is there to do? I had no control, as though I was just along for the ride—like being caught up in a tornado. I'll land wherever it puts me down. I just went on. It was Don who bore the worst of all that went on—living with the choices he did not make; results he didn't understand. I am a reasonable person. I tried to make sense of what Don's children did. I tried to find a reason or even an excuse for their actions, but I only came up with more questions: Did they not remember the past year? Did they think he was going to recover when they finally found a "miracle drug"? Did they think he was faking his illness? If not Lewy body, what did they think was wrong with him? Why would they put him through this suffering?

Did they ever think, "Oh my. This is what it was like for Carol."?

By the time I had permission to see Don, he was about to be released from the hospital and returned to the care home. I could not believe what I saw after ten days, when he returned to the home. His appearance was shocking. I literally thought he was going to die that very day. His tremors were so violent he could not stand, even with support. He slept all the time with his tongue rolled back into his throat, so dry the underside had slit open. His eyes were always partially opened. He had deep bedsores that were angry and oozing. I was told that in the two weeks he was in the Cuckoo's Nest, only one medication had been changed. That week and a half in the ward was devastating to him, and for no reason except to assuage Kate's desires. I kept saying over and over, senselessly, "What have they done to you?"

Finally, the "visitation plan" was presented to the court. It was disappointing, to say the least. I received a little bit of freedom in that it said we all must simply abide by whatever rules the care home imposed. It allowed me to bring in a drink or a snack for Don, like everyone else did. But I still could not take Don out of the home. Kate was to notify me by e-mail of any and all changes in Don's condition, medications, or venue. That was it. Privileges for me were not addressed. At that time, it was a moot point whether I could take Don out for ice cream because of his condition. But as the weeks went by, Don rallied and improved, and we were again in the daily game of a hundred ways to say no whenever I asked to take Don out. The caregivers intervened when they could and told Don that this was not my choice but that of his daughters. He didn't understand and became upset with me, and I would leave without him.

Crossing the Borders

Christmas Day, Don was being taken to Kate's for the day. The caregivers at the nursing home alerted me so that I could see him Christmas Eve; I could stay for as long as I wanted. I put my rose-colored glasses on and began to get excited as I imagined Christmas Eve around the tree at his home; he could open his gifts from me and we could just spend a wonderful evening together. Several years ago, I had given Don a new wedding ring. Since he could no longer have it, I had it sized for my hand, and I was anxious to show him the gift he was giving me.

When I arrived, Don lit up like the Christmas tree itself, and grinning from ear to ear, he hugged me as tight as he ever had. I was sure this night was going to be everything I had imagined! But after a moment, he changed and began to pace, faster and faster, around the house, first pulling me with him, and then dragging me behind him. He had become psychotic in an instant, and I was afraid. I put the gifts I had brought for everyone at the home under the tree and left in tears.

I saw Don for my two allotted hours every day. And that was enough. When he was well, he was bored and would get agitated and upset with everybody around him. When he was ill, he suffered and it broke my heart. And every day was different. I would sit quietly with Don and wait for him to speak as though he was confiding something in me. If I listened with my heart, I could hear what he was trying to tell me. Sometimes, he told me his secrets. Most of the time, there was no message there. He was in a world apart from mine, and he was lost in it. But I loved him, so I loved him. Sometimes, he would have a moment of clarity. Without any warning, he would come out of his fog of confusion and say passionately, "I miss you so much," and then the moment would be gone and so would he. And that was enough for me that day. I had to leave even if it made him angry or sad or accusatory. I couldn't make everything all right. I couldn't fix it. Sometimes, I had to just run away.

I walked out of the care home and everything seemed surreal. It was a strange feeling—like I was dead but hadn't left this earth. Everything was foggy and could disappear at any moment. Like the soul had gone out of the earth. As I looked out from inside me, things looked different, as though it was all pretend or like when I blurred my eyes and everything was slightly out of focus. That's what my days were like.

I bought Don an electric toothbrush, thinking it would be easier for him. Don was afraid of the new toothbrush. And maybe for the first time, it really sunk in that my smart, wise husband was insane; he was *afraid of a toothbrush.* To say the words; to realize their meaning; how could this be, that Don has lost his mind?

I had to learn to draw lines. When I walked into the nursing home, guilt came over me ... guilt for having a life outside these walls. When I walked out, I had to learn how to shut the door on that existence and not think of it until I walked through the doors again. If I thought about Don being alone and lonely, or not sleeping, or being confused and delusional, I could not contain my grief. He sat alone with nothing to do, nothing to occupy his time or mind. He sat with his legal pad and calculator, but he could not write and did not remember how to use the calculator. He couldn't watch television, and any noise upset him. He was in a surreal world all alone.

He talked of visits from his brother, who died years ago. Maybe he did visit him. Who am I to say our spirits do not communicate as transitions of life take place? Don lived in Purgatory—he was amongst neither the living nor the dead. He was without purpose, without process, without connection; in a prison, kept from his home and family, locked in a strange house with people who were unknowable, and who came and went without explanation. He had no interests, no activity—of the body or mind. He had nothing that belonged to him. Confusion even of his bodily needs dominated him. He couldn't sleep at night, so he ransacked his room. He couldn't stay awake during the day. He pulled shut the curtains of consciousness and retreated somewhere inside himself. I often saw him close his eyes and "go away" just to stop the noise of idle talk and nonsense. Once he sat at the table with his eyes tightly closed while I spoke to him. "You can't see me. I'm not here," he said almost in a whisper. And most of the time, when I spoke to him of something important, if he looked at me at all, he had a confused or agitated look on his face and didn't understand what I said. But once in a while, he answered me with clarity and deep emotion. I cherished those moments. For a little while, I got to believe again that we were who we used to be. As I helped him stand, I held him close to me. Although he seemed completely disinterested in my touch now, the closeness of him still stirred me. His body was still the tower I climbed into—it was where I felt safe and at peace.

Like the Eagles' *Hotel California*, in our world, *"You can check out any time you like, but you can never leave."*

What Was Meant for Evil

I have referred to a scripture in Genesis: "What was meant for evil, God will turn for good." And now I turn to what good has and will come from this time of my life.

First, it is a good thing that I am not the same person I was two years ago. I feel as though I was rather useless then. Don had spoiled me dreadfully, with love and with all the wonderful things love brings. Now I know about joy that is there in spite of circumstances; about love that transcends the physical; about patience and the goodness of taking care of the needs of another adult; about having friends and family that are dear; about faith and trust in God whose spirit goes through these times with us; about liking myself and finding purpose to my life; about teaching what I have learned. Nothing much bothers me now. It bewilders me how when something goes wrong (even a big dent in my little car), it just doesn't seem to matter, because I know in time, "all things work together." I bring calm and confidence to situations. I bring a measure of wisdom that I didn't have before. I listen better and have more compassion.

It is a good thing that I did not have to make the decisions regarding Don's medical treatment. Although I objected to many of the decisions Kate made, I didn't know what was right, so I was happy that I didn't carry that weight. I could walk out the door, close it, and not carry guilt or remorse.

This situation was a great learning process. Bankers, estate planners, members of blended families, same-sex partners, and older couples all have asked me for guidelines and advice. There are so many aging blended families now. In the hospitals where Don was treated, the social workers told me that in the last few years they had seen more of the type of conflict I experienced. Greed, perhaps. Jealously for love or closeness lost. Control. Whatever brings this action, there are some lessons that can be learned.

In my case, I came to believe that there were undercurrents long before February 11, 2007. I have always been so perceptive and intuitive that I sometimes even scared myself! Why had I not seen *this* coming? I look back now and I believe that Don's children were choosing to believe his delusions and were urging him to act on them months prior to February 11, 2007. I believe they were doing this out of jealousy of the love that Don and I shared and showed to each other. Possibly, they never really accepted me, so when their dad was so lost and confused, they came to think he had become disillusioned with me and were ready and waiting to rescue him from me. I think Carla put distrust in Don's mind. I think she must have used his confusion about the Carols and home to talk to him of divorce, even before Christmas. I think they became obsessed with the whole thought pattern after a while and were simply lost in their own delusions, losing all perspective. I think they wanted to punish me for curbing Frank, and they wanted Frank to have the Quarry. I think they thought we had more assets than we actually did. I think they were also afraid that if Don had the same disease as his brother (and there is reason to believe his father may also have suffered from it), that it might be hereditary, and by admitting that, they would admit to their own fate. By believing that his wife caused his suffering and it was not a disease, they were free from worry about themselves. Not one, *not one* of any of that family—not even Don's sister-in-law Iona, to whom both Don and I had been so close—ever supported me with even a telephone call. Doug's wife, who had known me longer than Don had known me, did not give me the benefit of a doubt.

I think Don's granddaughter, Amanda, told a false story about what happened the day I knocked on the door, which incensed the family and put them into a rage. While Don lived with Kate and her family, I believe this thirteen-year-old saw herself as Don's champion. From the time he returned to me in March 2007, she was at war with me for Don's attention and love. I hope someday she realizes what a needless war she fought.

Not for one moment do I think they actually believed the accusations they made.

I often wonder about the marriages of Don's children; they do not seem to understand loving one another. I have wondered how they can go to bed together and not think about themselves being separated against their will. I wonder how the parents explained this to their children. Most of the grandchildren were old enough to understand that there was animosity and bitterness in the family, and that Grandma and Grandpa were not together anymore. I cannot imagine what they were told. It reminded me of a story:

Once a frail old man went to live with his son, daughter-in-law, and four-year-old grandson. The old man's hands trembled, his eyesight was blurred and his step faltered. The family ate together at the table, but the elderly grandfather's shaky hands and failing sight made eating difficult. Peas rolled off his spoon onto the floor. When he grasped his glass, milk spilled onto the tablecloth.

The son and daughter-in-law became irritated with the mess. "We must do something about Father," said the son. "I've had enough of his spilled milk, noisy eating, and food on the floor." So the husband and wife set a small table in the corner. There, Grandfather ate alone while the rest of the family enjoyed dinner at the table. Since Grandfather had broken a dish or two, his food was served in a wooden bowl. When the family glanced in Grandfather's direction, sometimes he had a tear in his eye as he sat alone. Still, the only words the couple had for him were sharp admonitions when he dropped a fork or spilled food.

The four-year-old watched it all in silence. One evening before supper, the father noticed his son playing with wood scraps on the floor. He asked the child sweetly, "What are you making?" Just as sweetly, the boy responded, "Oh, I am making a little bowl for you and Mama to eat your food from when I grow up."

Whether it is karma, God's justice, or the world righting itself, I believe we reap what we sow. I believe that our children learn how to treat us by watching how we treat our parents. I believe we can curse our own lives and families by evil actions. I leave these things to God.

As for forgiveness, I leave that to God also. Many times, I struggled with my anger and wanted to pray for "the Big Bus" to come along! There were months when I couldn't bear to sit in Don's room and see the ever-present collage of smiling faces across from me on the wall. But after a while, I just quit feeling anything emotional about them at all. They were just people I had to deal with but for whom I had no emotional feeling, one way or the other. What they did, they did to their father. If and when they should ever ask for forgiveness, I will simply say, "You are asking the wrong person." I hold them accountable for what they have done, but I will not allow them to cause bitterness or malice or to define my character.

I'm not even sure I understand forgiveness. I have no power to forgive; I cannot exonerate anyone; how can one human stand in judgment of another? What I can do is to abdicate the desire to stand in judgment, to let my hurt feelings go, and to simply give that person to God to deal with. Since I have no power over another to either change him or to judge him, to continue to try to do so is to rob myself of time, energy, and peace.

March 2008

Every day, someone asked how Don was doing. I always had to consider how to answer; he had lost his mind. Lewy body dementia is an episodic disease, taking its victim through phases. For a few weeks, Don slept all the time, unable to awaken. Then he went through a few weeks where he could not sleep at all and became sleep deprived. He would be lethargic, and then so agitated that he had to be moving all the time. He hallucinated for a few weeks, and then he was as though he was in a coma. He changed.

After Don's last stay in the Cuckoo's Nest, he lost so much weight that he was a mere skeleton. His appetite was good, so I began to bring in a healthy egg breakfast sandwich each morning. He loved it, ate every bite, and asked for two, and he was ready for lunch when served! He began to put on weight, so it seemed like a good thing. It also seemed to solve the very real problem of his begging to go out with me. I often brought muffins for all of the residents, and every Sunday morning was "Doughnut Day," when I brought two dozen fresh, warm doughnuts for all the residents. In a nursing home, this is a treat, and it was welcomed and encouraged by the administrators of the home. Don looked forward to whatever I brought him each day and stood by the window waiting for me. The old adage "The way to a man's heart is through his stomach" was absolutely true for us; when he sometimes wasn't able to remember our marriage relationship, I settled for being "the doughnut lady."

Then he had severe edema. His feet and hands looked like "mitts." But after complete blood tests, no identifiable problem was found, so of course, the kids assumed that I was to blame. It must have been the foods that I brought in for Don. I received an e-mail message from Kate that said, "I'm requesting that all of Dad's visitors [I am a visitor!] refrain from bringing in food and drink, wrapped [or] unwrapped." We've been down this road before! Other relatives brought in hamburgers, fries, ice cream—everything … so this must have been about poisoning again.

I took my concern to the administrator. They thought surely that it was only meant to include anything that might be thought "salty," so I asked Kate if I was being restricted from the Sunday morning doughnuts. The reply was, "Please follow the directions as outlined in my original e-mail."

I would like to say I was not affected by this response. But I was. Not only was this a direct accusation, but it affected my time with my husband. This was *not* about poison, it was about hate. They did not believe I was sprinkling medications on doughnuts and serving them to all the residents, the caregiver, and myself. How could I explain to six patients with dementia that there would be no more Sunday morning doughnuts? How could I answer my husband when I came empty-handed to him in the morning? He would feel I was not meeting his needs and want to know why. We had precious little to talk about or spend our time doing together, and now I could look forward to his begging and his accusations again. In discouraging moments, I thought, *Maybe I should just not go anymore.* It was not a matter of me wanting to take food. It was a matter of doing something for him and the others that made them feel loved and special and that broke the terrible monotony.

Don was asleep when I entered his room one day. When I sat beside him, he opened his eyes and said, "Let's eat!" I had nothing to give him. We sat together as he kept asking for something to eat, and a tear rolled down his cheek. I wiped it away, and he said, "My heart is breaking. You don't love me anymore." My heart was breaking, too.

I made a plea to the attorney who had written the impotent visitation agreement, but received absolutely no response from her. I decided to stand with the original agreement and abide by the rules of the home, and continued to bring doughnuts. I risked "doughnut jail," from which friends pledged they would make bail in the event I was in any way punished for the doughnuts.

Doug came from Dallas. Don was agitated. He was very aware of what he was saying, and when I listened, he made perfect sense. He told me he wanted to go where we could talk alone; he asked about selling our land and was worried about me not getting what I should from the sale. He said *we* had bought it and planned for it to be for both of *us*. It became obvious that Doug was discussing every detail of conservancy with him again, and it was causing him great turmoil. There was no way for me to answer him. I told him it was all working out fine, and that I loved him. He said, "I love you more than a million …," and trailed off as his eyes welled. What was the denial of this despicable family doing to this poor, sweet man? I rethought my whole philosophy on forgiveness.

Lessons

Although many may experience Alzheimer's or dementia or another debilitating disease, which is in itself a horrible thing, most will not be faced with the hateful actions that I faced. My story was one where many unlikely things came together at once and created the "perfect storm." I believe that if there were not two attorneys in the family who knew how to get what they wanted, this action would never have taken place. Knowledge is power; and they had all the power. I believe most of what was done in this situation was simply "because they could." They knew the law and they knew how to make it work for them. Bill Clinton, who once said he did things "because he could," now calls that reasoning "the most morally indefensible reason that anybody could have for doing anything." For a moment, I like old Bill.

The lessons I have learned are practical, and not meant to be legal advice or taken as such. A lawyer may tell you, "That's not how the system works," but I am saying that the system did not work for me. Many times I did not even feel that my own lawyers were doing what was right for me, much less the court system. The judge's opinion that "it will all shake out in the end" did not work for me. I was not given my day in court to present my side, and the most I got out of the system was that the horrendous charges of attempting to kill my husband were dropped after I gave up all of our joint assets. It was nothing short of legal blackmail. They would press to the courts the bogus charges and would "dog her the rest of her life" if I did not agree to all of their demands.

What I offer here as lessons are simply practical things I learned to which everyone should take heed. Under ordinary circumstances, the following should protect you as the spouse, completely. Each of these documents can be challenged in court, but that is not the action commonly taken. To date I have $35,000 in legal fees, and the legal fees of Don's family are well over $50,000. Most families cannot and will not spend that kind of money on challenging legal documents that are in place.

- PREPARATIONS

1. The most important thing of all is to have a durable power of attorney and a medical power of attorney in place. There are many degrees of powers of attorney with different directives. A durable POA allows a designated person to fulfill all legal duties just as though you were performing them yourself. It extends through your lifetime, even through incompetency. It is automatically revoked at death. A medical POA gives a designated person the power to make medical decisions for you in your stead. Neither of these documents require an attorney or filing of record. They must be notarized and kept for presentation when required.

Neither of these documents kept Don's children from challenging them in the ex parte order. Most people will not be faced with such an extreme act; therefore, your POAs can be the most important documents you can have as a spouse. Being married does not automatically give you authority in a world of the Privacy Act of 1974. If a wife makes a call inquiring about an insurance policy held by her husband, even if she is the beneficiary, she will not be given any information without a copy of his power of attorney. Not even a mailing address can be changed for your spouse without a power of attorney. Inquiries about bills, credit cards, or phone service that is in the spouse's name cannot be accessed without a power of attorney. However, if someone other than the spouse holds a POA, they have access to all of the personal documents and privileges *to the exclusion of the spouse.* The person to whom you grant durable power of attorney should be someone you trust with every penny you have in the world, because that is what they have access to.

2. Set up a revocable trust. Setting up a trust changes ownership. Property put into a trust belongs to the trust and is no longer subject to probate if the individual dies. You may still have control of the assets put into a revocable trust by remaining the trustee of the trust. I chose a simple revocable trust whereby I am the trustee and can amend the trust at any time before my death. My "Family Trust" transfers all of the assets of the trust (whatever I choose to deed in the name of the trust) to my son and his children, bypassing probate. A Pour Over will is usually made a part of the trust, transferring all properties not specifically listed in the trust to the trust. No one but the trustee can amend the trust. If properties that are to be transferred into the trust are in joint tenancy, the other party has to sign the deed over, or his POA can sign for him, so it is imperative that this action be taken either before incapacity, or while the spouse has a valid POA.

A living trust can also make a very effective prenuptial agreement. Any property you put into your living trust before you marry remains the property of that trust and stays separate from property accumulated during your marriage—even in community property states. It is not uncommon to have three living trusts in one family—each spouse has a separate living trust for property acquired before the marriage (usually giving it to their respective children from a previous marriage), and the couple has a joint living trust for property acquired during the marriage.

States vary regarding tenancy laws, so the best course of action is to confer with an attorney or estate planner to be sure of the best way to protect yourself in your state. However, a trust is not a recorded document. The only requirements are signature notarization, and the transference and recording of deeds to the trust. (These documents are under state jurisdiction, so each state may have some unique language and requirements. You should make sure the documents are correct for your state.)

Because I did not have a trust before Don's illness and the resulting conflict, I was advised that the act of transferring properties into a trust would not protect them from Don's children if we went to trial. However, I thought at the very least it would slow them down a little. They could sue me for the assets transferred into the trust (which they did), stating that I had "gifted assets belonging to Don" and thus breached my fiduciary responsibilities. A court would have had to agree that I did that with the intention of taking property from Don. I believe they did not pursue this action because I proved that the properties I put in the trust were not Don's properties but mine, individually. Had those properties not been tied up in a trust, I have no doubt the children would have included my home and rental property in the lawsuit, along with our joint properties. (A revocable living trust will never protect assets. The principle is that if you can get to your assets, then so can a valid creditor. In order to protect assets from creditors, the trust would have to be irrevocable and funded prior to knowledge of an impending claim. Otherwise, it would be considered a "fraudulent transfer.")

In the summer of 2009, Byrd and Melanie Billings, parents of sixteen children (twelve of whom were adopted, special-needs children), were murdered. Instead of protecting her family with a trust, Mrs. Billings had a will. Her adult daughter stepped in to take over the care of the nine minor children, acting to immediately have the will settled so she could house and support the children. *According to Florida law*, a will must be witnessed by two people, under specific conditions. It turned out that documentation of the will's witnesses was not properly executed; therefore, the will was not recognized. Mrs. Billings was considered "intestate." Money was not available to the family, and her estate became subject to probate. *Before entering into any legal document, be sure to check your state's requirements and adhere to them in detail.*

3. Prepare a living will. A living will is a document that states one's wishes concerning end-of-life decisions. Don always said he wanted to "go nose to the pavement," meaning he wanted to die instantly. Of course, we all do. We do not want to suffer or live a life without quality. When Don became incapacitated, it was too late for him

to express his wishes. They were not thought through and written down, so he was at the mercy of whoever had control over his medical treatment. The result was that Don's children could decide to keep him alive indefinitely with a feeding tube or dialysis. Living wills, like powers of attorney, are state controlled. As an example, California has a statutory document for use as a living will. At the end of this book, I have included a copy of my personalized living will, simply a letter to my family emphasizing my end-of-life decisions to go along with my formal end-of-life directive.

- JOINT ACCOUNTS AND JOINT TENANCY

1. Almost all married couples have joint banking accounts. In our marriage, Don and I had our separate personal banking accounts, separate business accounts, and separate savings and investment accounts. However, it seemed prudent to have both names on each account for reasons of accessibility in the event of death or injury, not to mention trust in the marital relationship. Don did not carry checks for my checking accounts, nor did I carry checks for his, but we did know they were accessible to us if need be, as we were both signers on all of the accounts. This turned out to be very important when Don became unable to pay his personal bills and carry on the daily business of his management company. I was able to write checks on these accounts without any confusion or delay, which was of paramount importance.

However, it was these joint accounts that Carla accessed and from which she took all the money with a signed power of attorney for Don. His POA was able to take all of the money out of all of these accounts without notifying me, and she did. This can also be done by either of the joint owners of the accounts in the case of separation or divorce. The bank says it is "whoever gets there first."

Since this is the way the bank does business, we must educate ourselves as to the rules. My suggestion would be to keep as little money in joint accounts as is necessary. All money over the necessary amounts to do business should be moved to personal, solely owned accounts. If a POA is in place for the spouse, checks can be signed using the POA. In our case, this meant that, if need be, Don could have signed my personal checks, but no one *else* could have gained access to my accounts through him.

Most financial documents offer a Payment on Death (POD) or Transfer on Death (TOD) option. This is offered on deeds, bank accounts, savings accounts, security accounts, and so on. The owner designates one to whom the funds will be made available *upon the death of the owner*. The beneficiary does not have joint ownership of the account, but ownership is transferred to them without probate upon proof of death. Always take advantage of this option. POD can allow your spouse (or whomever you choose) to access all funds upon your death and is an option to joint tenancy. This is particularly effective when a surviving parent is leaving funds to children, wants to avoid probate, but doesn't want to make assets accessible to the child's creditors. No form is required other than the designation with the financial institution.

2. When dealing with real estate, there are several ways in which it can be held. A married couple usually holds property in joint tenancy with right of survivorship (JTWROS). This method gives each spouse (or owner) one half of the property and at the death of one spouse (or owner), his or her ownership transfers to the surviving spouse (or owner). JTWROS does not allow for the property to be *inherited*. In other words, when Don dies, his half of the property goes directly to me and will not be a part of his estate or inherited by his children. Our joint assets were set up this way because it was the intent of us both that the properties be *ours*, for our benefit.

Tenants in common involves individual interests in group ownership. Each owner may have a different percentage of interest in the whole property. Upon the death of one of the owners, the interest *is* inheritable. Unmarried partners would probably want to use this type of ownership so that each of their heirs would inherit their percentage interest.

My husband and I chose joint tenancy with right of survivorship. Don's children could not sell these properties or take over the properties with this type of ownership. Without my participation, the properties could not be touched. Due to the lawsuit, I agreed to issue a quit claim deed to Don's conservancy so that they could sell the property. Otherwise, they would have no claim to any of our properties.

We held the Quarry in a limited liability partnership, because as its name suggests, liability (lawsuits or damages) is limited to the investment you have in the partnership. The nature of the Quarry—being a recreation property on the water—presented considerable financial risk. Don and I each owned 50 percent of the property; therefore, we were the only partners. As above, Don's children could not sell or take over this property. I would remain a partner until I resigned or gave a quit claim to the property; however, at Don's death, his 50 percent would go into his estate. Again, due to the lawsuit, I agreed to resign in favor of Don's conservancy.

3. When dealing with vehicle ownership, generally a husband and wife hold the title as "and/or." In this case, one of the spouses can sell the vehicle without the signature of the other. Don and I owned my car and his truck this way. Had Don's children been able to get the Cadillac title (which they could have with Don's POA by requesting a duplicate title), they could have sold it without my knowledge or signature. I knew this, so in order to protect my vehicle, I traded the car, which was in both our names as "and/or," and put my new car in my name only. In this way, I protected my car from his kids taking possession of it. I respected his truck as his property, and when I turned it over to his kids, I simply gave them the title so they could sell it at will without my participation. The positive side to "and/or" ownership is that if one spouse dies or becomes incapacitated (without a durable power of attorney), the remaining spouse can sell the vehicle without going through probate. The other remedy is to place the vehicle in your trust.

- <u>CASH AND PERSONAL POSSESSIONS</u>

1. Cash. The history of our case, where Carla took our cash from the various bank accounts, was scary enough. I didn't feel there was anything safe anywhere from her. She had simply taken Don with her into the banks, armed with his power of attorney, and asked for

any and all accounts attached to his Social Security number, and the money was handed over. As soon as I was aware of this action, I opened new accounts in my name only. But within a short period of time, their attorneys demanded copies of my personal accounts. They were poised to take everything they could from my accounts. During this time, I was concerned that the court would "freeze" my accounts pending a trial, and I would not have access to my own money. I asked how I could protect my money; could I convert to cash? My attorney said the court would see through the bank statements that I had converted money to cash, and it probably would not be protected.

However, I had learned enough to put protecting what I had first. If my accounts were frozen, I would have no recourse. I took what money I had in my accounts and converted the sum to a cashier's check. That cashier's check could not be touched by anyone but me without a court order, but it was accessible to me. Then, as my income came in, I would cash my checks and begin to accumulate cash and keep only what was necessary to pay my monthly bills in my checking accounts. I knew that if and when the kids and their attorneys looked at my personal accounts, any withdrawals would be questioned, so every time I went to the grocery or shopping center, I wrote the check for the maximum over the purchase amount and kept the extra cash in my "sock under the mattress." By the time we finally reached a settlement and my assets were no longer threatened, I had saved several thousands of dollars in this manner. It gave me great security to know that my income was not in jeopardy during this time.

2. Personal property. At one time, we had a small antique store. The years that Don and I auctioned, we had the opportunity to buy rare, small antiques to sell in the store. We had several storage sheds full of items and also stored many things in our home, and we had an abundance of antiques in our home. During this time, we insured these possessions for $50,000 as personal property. Among these antiques were quite a bit of antique jewelry. We put the insured amount of $50,000 on our financial statement. Don's children got a copy of our financial statement from the bank for those years, and

they wanted me to pay them $25,000 for Don's half of our personal property. This was beyond surprising to me! We had closed the shop many years earlier, sold off all remaining antique items, moved and changed our décor, and downsized considerably from our Victorian antique days. I had to go through my house and put a value on every item in our home to show that we had nowhere near that amount in personal possessions now, and in the process, I noted that I had paid for every item in our home out of my income, not Don's. Don brought the usual divorced man's fare into our marriage (a recliner, a television set, and a desk), while I had a full house of furnishings. The lesson here is to guard against such misinformation and keep good records of what you have and how you got it.

After Don was in the nursing home and I knew he would never come back to our home, I went on a cleaning jag! I wanted to get rid of extra baggage we had accumulated and to simplify; to get the things that no longer had purpose or that I was not particularly attached to out of my life. First, I removed every picture of Don's family from my home. These people were not my family any longer, and I did not want to see their smiling faces in my house. As I cleaned closets and drawers, I took every reminder of them and put everything in a box. I put the shabby clothes that I had removed from Don's rooms in the box. I put Don's personal mementos from his childhood and from his parents in the box. Things that were his personally, to which I had no attachment, I put in the box for his children to keep. At one time, no one was interested in his family history or the documents and pictures passed down from his grandparents, but I made a scrapbook of these things that the kids had admired. I put the pages in the box. Gifts that they had given him went into the box. One box overflowed and became two and then three. I kept the things that were meaningful to Don and me, and to which I had an attachment. Pictures of Don are still everywhere in our home, and to see them is comforting. They fill the rooms with his presence. This is still our home together, and he belongs here.

When Doug came to collect Don's truck and his guns, I made sure he took the boxes, which would be the last tangible sign of any relationship between Don's children and me.

3. Make sure you understand your rights as a surviving spouse. I have heard heartbreaking stories of women being put out of the home they shared with their husband because the husband's children took possession and convinced her she had no rights to anything. In Kansas, a law was passed that provides if a man and woman were married a certain number of years and one died, the survivor is entitled to a minimum percentage of the combined augmented estate. The percentage is graduated until, after fifteen years of marriage, it reaches one half the total value of assets. This law was passed because there were a lot of second and third marriages, some of which had lasted many, many years, and the will left out the survivor completely, sometimes leaving the surviving spouse nearly destitute. The surviving spouse has four months to file a claim against the estate for the share for which she may be entitled. If she does not file in time, she forfeits the right to the share she would otherwise receive. This is an area where you need to see an attorney immediately following the death of your spouse, who can inform you of the laws in your state.

- <u>PRACTICAL EVERYDAY LESSONS</u>

1. Thankfulness. Recently I took a class called "An Introduction to Judaism for the Non-Jew." The teaching of the rabbi awed me in the first session as he spoke about the very detailed and disciplined practices of Judaism in everyday life. One of their objectives is to thank God for *one hundred things every day*, from the gift of life upon awakening, to the gift of sleep at night. I began to practice thankfulness. I thanked God for everything that came my way, including the things I did not like. Instead of blessing the food at mealtime, I followed the Jewish pattern and blessed God for the food. Every time I expressed thankfulness, I was praying. What a difference in my attitude and outlook this made! Counting our blessings is not a new concept, but it is one that seems to have been

lost along our way. I believe it is a necessary part of overcoming the adversities in our life.

2. Write it down. I mentioned my four-inch-thick journal, which was entered into court records. I am sure that Don's children found it more entertaining than effectual, but it recorded every day from the onset of Don's illness and of his decline. It recorded every action and conversation that took place between Don's family, Don, and me. It held every e-mail that went between us. Many times when I was asked to recall a certain date or certain happenings, I could not do it without going back and looking in my journal. Many accusations were made that were easily disproved by referring to the facts in my journal. Had we gone before a judge or jury, this written information would have become vital to proving my innocence of all charges.

3. The legal system. I do not pretend to know much about our legal system—except what has happened to me. Inevitably, when people would hear that Don was taken out of our home and isolated from me, they would say, "They can't do that!" They referred to "the law" and "the rights" that we have under our laws. That is like saying to the bank robber, "You can't do that." Yes, he can. The rapist "can." The murderer "can." And when they do, it is then up to the injured party to bring them to accountability. *The law itself does not keep anyone from doing anything.* What Don's children did to him was against our laws and our sense of decency, but that did not keep them from doing it. I think we should be clear minded about our legal system. *Anyone can do anything to anybody*; had I wanted in the beginning to sue them, I could have. Eventually, they turned the tables on me, claiming that they were the injured party and sued me, leaving me the one to prove my innocence.

In April of 2008, 440 children, from infants to teenagers, were removed from their parents and home in a raid on the Yearning for Zion Ranch in Eldorado, Texas, by ex parte order. This action was the result of an *anonymous* phone call with nothing more to back up accusations than suspicion and prejudice. It was later determined that the call was a *hoax* made by a thirty-three-year-old Colorado woman who had no relationship at all with the Ranch. It resulted in these children being separated from their home and parents for over a year, at a cost to the government of $14 million. On June 2, 2009, almost all of the children were returned to their parents and the cases dropped due to the lack of cause for the action. The courts may say, "It all shakes out in the end," but at what cost and damage to the children and their families? The laws need to be changed so that some substantial proof is a requirement for as serious an action as an ex parte order. This is a reflection of decent human values being affected by out-of-control legal system professionals.

Navigating through the world of attorneys is another problem. They are a requirement of the system and a necessity because the layperson has no idea how this game is played. *And it is a high-stakes "game."* Most of the time I felt my attorneys were more interested in keeping the opposing attorneys happy than with doing or saying what I needed. I wanted—needed—a champion. I wanted to feel someone was on my side, an advocate who was committed to my welfare alone, and I rarely felt that. This was my life and my future they had in their hands, but they had many cases going at once, and mine really wasn't that lucrative for them. As with doctors, you have to be proactive with your case and insist that they follow up or make things happen. In my case, *depositions* were expensive, time consuming, emotionally draining, frightening, and pointless, and they served only to intimidate. After my long deposition, I asked for a copy of the transcript. Surprisingly, I found that although a court reporter was paid to take down every word, every sigh, it would cost another $400 to have it transcribed and made available, and that was never done.

4. Medicaid. If Don lived long enough, eventually the money in his conservancy account would have been used up. If that time came, the financing of his care would have been my responsibility as his spouse, by law. I would not have the income to finance his nursing home care. Medicaid (not to be mistaken for Medicare) would pay for long-term nursing home care. To start Medicaid coverage, certain financial criteria must be met, but you can still hold certain assets. No attempt is made to recover medical costs until the death of the person who received benefits. The Estate Recovery program is then

used to recover assets owned by a deceased person who received medical coverage. Estate Recovery attorneys will file a claim against a deceased person's estate (assets subject to probate) to collect for medical bills Medicaid paid. They only recover money after funeral expenses are paid. If there are no assets left, they do not ask for money back. In Kansas, if the Medicaid recipient has a surviving spouse, recovery is delayed until the death of the spouse (however, this depends on the jurisdiction—state by state and even, to some extent, county by county). Medicaid will recover most assets in which the recipient has an ownership interest. For example, they will recover from assets such as life insurance proceeds, life estates (not to be confused with a revocable trust), trust funds, and jointly owned property. They can also recover assets conveyed upon death through special deeds and titles, such as a transfer on death deed or tenancy in common. *The homestead is exempt until the death of the surviving spouse*, but the state may place a lien on the home to recover what they pay out for nursing home care. The home would be sold after the death of the surviving spouse, satisfying the lien. The state can only recover from assets owned by the recipient and not from assets owned by the spouse of the recipient. Obviously, as you are reading this, you might wonder what you could do to get your homestead and any other assets out of your name so you would not be subject to the Medicaid recovery. However, Medicaid goes back *three to five years* to check for retitled or sold properties. My suggestion is that you plan far ahead and take into consideration the Medicaid rules so that your properties can be legally diverted into trusts or transferred to heirs long before this time comes. If you have assets, this is one area where money spent on an estate attorney would be money well spent.

 The irony of my situation was that being Don's spouse, I was legally responsible for his care throughout his life. We had sufficient assets to sell that would pay for long-term care, including my personal properties and personal money (until it was gone), to sustain Don. If the assets had been used up, then Medicaid would have been there for us. What a profane use of the last two years and the tens of thousands of dollars spent on attorneys for nothing.

5. Take care of yourself. The Alzheimer's Association says that *60 to 80 percent of caregivers die before their spouse*, which is astounding! The stress of being Don's caregiver brought me to the doctor's office with severe stress, heart arrhythmia, and other serious physical problems including hemorrhaging, caused by lifting Don. It took me a long time to realize that Don needed more than I could give him, and that taking care of him could have taken my life.

One of the most difficult decisions we may have to make is *when* to place our loved one in nursing care. During my generation, that of the baby boomers, nursing homes had a very bad reputation. Our parents cried out, "Don't put me in one of those places!" A lot of guilt was attached to putting a loved one in a nursing home, so it is a difficult decision for us to come to. I wanted to keep Don at home—where I thought he would be most comfortable and would be cared for by someone who loved him, not strangers. I could not understand why keeping Don at home was not the best choice for him. When he could not be left alone, I put him in day care, but he fought against that so badly that I was riddled with guilt and could not even think of the day when he would have to go away from home for good.

The concept of nursing homes has changed much in the last decade. If you choose carefully, a very nice home can be found, as I have described. The thing I want to address now is *when* that decision should be made. Don's decline was so rapid and extreme that I waited too long. I have learned that when dementia sets in, "home" has no meaning. There is no memory of "home," and the place they have lived for years holds no comfort for them. In fact, the confusion is so prevalent that they seem to find comfort in a small room that has few objects or furniture; they require structure and direction. Meals need to be at a certain time each day. Believe me, in Don's care home, if lunch was one minute past twelve o'clock, the residents were all pounding the table! They could not remember whether they had breakfast or not, but they knew when it was time for lunch! They need someone caring for them who is not emotionally invested in them. Someone they cannot hurt with their words or actions, and cannot traumatize with their psychosis.

Incontinence with the inability to participate in one's own maintenance is one of the absolute signs that *it is time*. This person we love is an adult, not a baby. Especially women would like to think we can do this, but it is not something that endears either the caregiver or the patient. Although we want to be brave enough to take care of their personal needs, we are neither trained for nor capable of the demands. Think of when you have been in the hospital how, because it was the duty of the nurse, and it was impersonal, you were not embarrassed to allow the nurse to take care of your personal needs. It seemed that way with Don. He retained more dignity if I was not involved in those intimacies. And for me, being relieved of that responsibility was a great relief.

Don sometimes threw a little fit when I left him at the home each day. He even tried to run out the door with me, which ruined my day! I drove away thinking of him sitting in his room alone with my picture, crying and kissing it! The truth was the nursing home had become his home and the people there, his family. As soon as the door was closed, he resumed his routine and forgot who I even was. And I could drive away knowing that he was being cared for and his every need was being met, and I could live! So I think it is usually the family that is not ready for the nursing home, not the one who is ill.

In extreme cases, our loved one may scream they want to go home and complain that they are being abused and starved in the home. It is the disease that is crying out, not the person we love. Dementia robs its victim of every sense; of reason; of memory. Many times the residents of Don's home, Don included, would tell me they had not been fed breakfast, or they had not eaten for days. Of course they had, but they were not expressing needs or rational thinking. Time after time, I watched the professional caregivers deal with these cries in an unemotional way that calmed the people. Stick around the home long enough to see these things for yourself, and then you will not feel the guilt or worry when you are not there.

I learned lessons every single day from Don. He was still my mentor. All the things this wonderful man always was, he was still, only more so. With his mind muddled and confused, still he was a gentleman who stood, wobbling, while he stepped aside for a lady to pass before him. He still would not sit before all of the ladies were seated. He still tried to pull out a chair and seat me at the table before himself. If I did not have a plate, he offered me everything on his before he ate for himself. He was grateful for everything and always expressed his appreciation. He was very tender and didn't hide his tears if something touched his heart. He readily apologized if he thought he had offended anyone. Sometimes he said he was so sorry, and I had no idea what he could be sorry for. He kept his sense of humor, dry as it was. The smile began around his eyes and then spread to his cheeks and lips when I laughed with him. He was loving to everyone, quick to give winks or touches to his housemates, and took every opportunity to help them in any way he could. He said to his housemates at the table, "It is most important that we keep our dignity." At times he seemed to grasp his plight and he confided, "It just isn't worth it anymore," but he kept on going. He did what was expected of him, and he didn't complain.

Special relationships are formed in the nursing home. There was a woman who was 103 years old who believed she knew Don in her past and they had been reunited. She watched over Don, and he was her special friend. He winked at her as he passed and lovingly patted her shoulder. Don was the dignitary of the little group; they all seemed to look to him for cues and responses. But they came and went, taken to the hospital or mortuary in the dark of night.

Don's philosophies were always pretty simple. He felt there was little else for which we were on earth if not to help one another. In our early years of marriage, we agreed that if we could change, I mean *really change*, the life of only one person in our lifetimes, we would have been successful. Don changed the lives of many. His faith was simple; he believed that if one knew God, he would do good. Once he listened quietly to my long dissertation of what Christianity was all about. At last he spoke: "If I do good, I feel good. If I do bad, I feel bad. So I do good." How simple is that? Don said we all come into this world with a wagon. In our wagon are a predetermined number of bricks that we must take through life with us. How we handle that load of bricks is the measure of who we are. Some will put their bricks in someone else's wagon to lighten their own load. Some will stop and pick up bricks that have been left by the wayside where they should be left; and some will lighten another's load when they feel strong. Don and I would often describe our day in terms of what happened with our bricks that day.

Don always said, "If Carol ever leaves me … I'm going with her!" (I think he stole the line from Kirk Douglas, but he believed it was his!) If there is one thing in this life I am sure of, it is that Don loved me completely. For that, I have been blessed beyond measure. I have been loved and romanced the way most women can only fantasize. At the nursing home, I was known as the "hot wife" (operative words here: *nursing home*), and Don was proud of me. He was very aware of who I was and what my role was in his life. He met me at the door when I came each day as though he'd been waiting for me. In a childlike way, he begged me to stay with him so we could be together. He would not even go to the bathroom without me for fear I would not be there when he came out. And yet, I had to leave each day. It broke my heart to leave him. I went to our home alone, and we both mourned a marriage torn from us against our wills.

Death Do Us Part

My husband died in the early morning hours of May 19, 2008. The death certificate says he died of "cardiac arrest as a consequence of metabolic acidosis as a consequence of coronary artery disease." The immediate cause of death was an abdominal aneurysm.

One day in April, I had again arrived at Don's home and found him gone, taken by ambulance in the early morning hours. No one could, or would, tell me what had happened; why he had been taken to the hospital; whether he was in serious condition; or to what hospital he was taken. Once again I was waiting for some word of whether my husband was dead or alive; sick or hurt. Kate told me nothing at all for over twenty-four hours. I finally received her e-mail telling me he was in the hospital after a fall, but she said they didn't want me to see him for a couple of days; she would not give me the hospital name or room number. I was becoming as resigned to this treatment as one in prison who has no control over her comings and goings. As soon as I was permitted, I went to the hospital and turned into the designated room, where I found the bed empty and neatly made up. At that moment of deep emotion, I felt out of my body; as though I were watching this frightened, confused little girl wondering if her beloved had died, or if this was just another mean, senseless lack of consideration. At the nurses' station, I found that Don had become very ill in the night and been taken to intensive care, and of course, they didn't even know he had a wife. When I saw him, I was taken back by his labored breathing, heaving chest, and pallor of death. Long seconds passed with his chest heaving up and down but he took no breaths. Finally, like a cannon going off unexpectedly, he forced air into his lungs. He was obviously near death that morning, and at his bedside, the doctors talked to me about resuscitation. Kate had ordered life support if necessary but the doctors were highly against that. Kate walked in during that conversation, and as I, Don's wife, stood right beside her, she told the doctors she would be conferring with her siblings and *they* would make a decision. The doctor looked at me with surprise, asked if I were not his wife, and said to me that he would not recommend resuscitation (as though I had any power!). This was the first time Kate and I had seen each other for a year. I could not stand her presence. I could not share space with the intruders who had stolen body and spirit from us. As I left the room, I asked Kate to give me specific hours I could be with Don without any of them present, and told her I would be back when they were not going to be there. Don lay near death being poisoned from acute renal failure—the very thing I had been accused of causing a year ago. I asked Kate, "Who are you going to blame now?"

Don recovered enough to be moved out of ICU, but he had failed significantly. He was too weak to move his own body, so he lay deathly still in the bed. He was comatose most of the time—totally unresponsive; however, every hour or so he would awaken for a few minutes and then return to his comatose state. I waited by his bedside for those minutes when he would wake and speak a few words, or eat a bite. On the third day, he opened his eyes and recognized me completely. He beckoned me to the bed, and I saw in his eyes the passion he had for me in the past. He put his arms around me and pulled my head onto his chest. He kissed me. As difficult as it was for his arms to do what he wished them to do, he brushed the hair from my eyes. He said quietly, "What a mess we are in." He asked if I was well; how was my health; was I alone; how did I get along. Although not everything he asked made sense, he was asking me if I was all right without him. He began to speak with expediency and said he may not be here tomorrow to tell me these things. He then began to tell me how much he had loved me and that I had been the most important person in his life. He held me, which he had not been able to do for months, and kissed me, and his eyes were full of the passion and love I had seen so many times before in our bed together. He said many things to me that day that will sustain me for the rest of my life. We were embraced in our passion for about forty-five minutes before he was forced back to the silence and darkness of his other world.

This hour of clarity and love frightened me as much as it fulfilled me. I had heard that sometimes people miraculously rallied just before death. These were moments, however, that I will cherish forever. I had not expected to ever have another chance to really share love with Don again.

Don lingered but after that day, he had few cognitive moments. He seemed so old and decrepit that he might just fade away with the next breath. He breathed laboriously, otherwise he did not move. Occasionally his legs scuffed against the sheets as though they were going somewhere, and his arms flailed into the air as though he was reaching for something, or shooing something away. He did not move any other part of his body, not even his head.

Eventually, he was moved to a higher level nursing home; a strange home, where he was just one of the ghosts that haunted the house. He was one of the bodies whose soul had gone on, but who could not die. Little rag dolls, they lay here or there, waiting … to be set free. The television was on, but no eyes were open to watch. A radio droned on, but no one could make out the words. It seemed it was only noise. The lot of them seemed to be comatose, and my husband was one of them, lost somewhere between life and death. Here, you believe in ghosts; spirits who cannot go to their resting place, yet were cursed to woefully walk among the living until some criteria was met.

I knew it would be a traumatic change for Don to be in a new environment, but I wasn't prepared for it to be traumatic for me. I had no say in where Don was put, of course. I just went where he was, following him wherever these people dictated for us both.

I didn't want Don in this home; I panicked; it made me ill to see him in this place. So much noise; no peace and no quiet. One man followed us every step we took, constantly making loud staccato sounds that Don thought were gunshots. The man never quit "ta-ta-ta-ta-ta-ta-ta-ing" on our heels, following us into Don's room and even the bathroom. How Don could control himself was a mystery, because I was fighting tears and the urge to push this human Uzi away. I needed him to stop the incessant noise, and I was sorry for Don that this was his life and he did not have any power over it. Don's body was broken, but his mind was not like the others; he was thinking and feeling, and he could be very articulate at times. Why was he there with people who could not think or feel? I wanted to scream, "Enough!" and take him home where he could live in peace and with love.

> *I could do it. I could bring him home. I could have two aides around the clock for the price of the nursing home. He could be in his own home with peace and quiet. Why can't I do this? If not my home, then he could go to Kate's with the aides. I would agree not to see him again if he could just be away from that asylum. Why can't we do this for Don?* (from my journal)

I e-mailed Kate and asked if she would consider other care for Don. But I was just like a barking dog in the neighborhood that is an annoyance and must be shut up.

My visits were not welcomed; apparently, these caregivers had been warned about me by Kate and Carla. Don's eyes were lost and vacant as though he was relentlessly searching for something he was doomed never to find. Most of the time, I don't think he knew who I was, only that I was someone who might help him as he groped his way toward something familiar in the heavy fog.

On Sunday afternoon, May 18, Don had a seizure and ceased to breathe. Kate ordered CPR until the ambulance arrived, and then they spent two more hours trying to revive him. He was coded for two and half hours.

I received a call from Carla that Sunday evening telling me only that Don was in the neuro-critical unit of the hospital. When I arrived, I found him on life support, violently convulsing every two to three minutes. His eyes were open, unresponsive, and clouded over. The doctors told me that as a result of being coded for two and half hours, his brain was damaged and his body was beginning to acidize, which means he was beginning to deteriorate. He was dead. The doctors asked me if I could talk sense to his children so he could be taken off life support. I told them I had no influence at all, but surely they would change their minds if they saw him in this condition.

The three of his children and his granddaughter, Amanda, who were at the hospital, were called in to see him. It was another out-of-body experience as I felt myself looking down on this odd gathering of people who all loved the same man. Kate seemed to be totally unmoved by his plight; her daughter, Amanda, would watch the harsh spasms of his seizures and say, "Grandpa is trying to sit up" or "Grandpa is trying to talk to us." No one corrected her. Carla was obviously upset by what she saw. Dennis, Don's youngest, stood across the room and stared at the floor. The doctors once again explained Don's condition, and Kate adamantly said she was going to leave him on life support for twenty-four hours longer to see if he improved and then make a decision. Twenty-four hours of convulsions. Twenty-four more hours on a respirator. I could not bear to watch my husband's life end in this desecration. He had finally reached the gateway of escape from Purgatory only to be barred entry into eternity for twenty-four more hours. I kissed his lips, and his skin was cold and as hard as the bone beneath it.

As I kissed my husband for the last time, Amanda looked down at me with her arms folded across her chest, with a look that made me shudder. She said, with narrowed eyes and intense hatred, "I am closer to him than you are!"

Although I said nothing and walked silently out of the door, my thoughts were, *You can crawl into that casket with him, baby, for all I care.*

After promising to call me immediately if anything changed, Kate did not call me until five hours after Don was taken off the respirator and pronounced dead. I waited all day and all evening to hear where they had taken his body. I tried to phone them in the evening, but they would not answer my calls. I was growing panicky to know where my husband's body had been taken. Late that evening, I called the hospital, hoping they would tell me which mortuary had picked up his body. They did. I called the mortuary to make an appointment to see him in the morning. I was told they had picked up his body early that morning, but no family member had contacted them all day concerning any arrangements. Once more, he lay all alone when I could have been with him.

I was, once again, in this final time of my life with my husband of eighteen years, being shut out of even burying him. When I met with the funeral director, I briefly explained the family situation and told him as Don's wife, I asked but a few things. I asked to be acknowledged as Don's wife in his obituary; I asked for my son and Rob's children to be acknowledged. I asked that I be allowed to approve the arrangements. These things were granted me. When I was called to approve the arrangements, I learned that even though I would be paying for the funeral, I was not to be given any input at all on the minister or have any part in the planning of the service. I was shown the casket. The kids had no minister in mind, so the funeral director referred one. In a strange coincidence, it was the hospice chaplain who had been present when Don was taken from our home by ex parte order last May. Not surprisingly, he was rejected. I brought Don's burial clothes to the funeral home and a picture for his obituary.

I was *never* contacted by Don's family regarding where he was, the funeral, or burial arrangements. I was told by the funeral director that Don was to be taken to a cemetery in Oklahoma for burial, but no arrangements were made for me. The funeral director saw to it that I was allowed first viewing of his body and all the time that I wanted to be with him privately, which I appreciated and of which I took great advantage.

The funeral was scheduled for Friday, May 23, at 10:00 am. There beside the casket was that same ever-present collage of pictures to shadow him, even in death. I was seated with the rest of the guests *behind* the family. As I sat from behind and looked over the "family," there were distant cousins of Don's, there was the mother of an in-law, there was a divorced daughter-in-law, there was Iona, and there was Frank, sitting next to his mother; but Don's wife of eighteen years was not among them. Frank, whom Don was afraid of and who was still actively pursuing his lawsuit against Don and me, was given the honor of pall bearer.

I sat amongst my family and the many friends that Don and I had enjoyed together over the years. As I looked at each face and saw their sorrow, I remembered the many times when Don and I shared something special with each one. The minister was a stranger to us all. The kids had met with him for an evening of stories and to get acquainted, and the eulogy simply related a few memories of childhood experiences. Doug then took the podium to tell a few more stories of their childhood; the stories were about the children and how their father had made them the successes they were now, not about Don. There was no mention of Don's personality or traits or the wonderful things he did for others or of his simple yet profound philosophies that changed people's lives. There was no mention of the many young people whom he had helped to start their own businesses, or those he had given work when no one else would hire them, to whom he taught work ethics. There was no mention of the healing he brought to the men who were in depression as he once was. Many of these people were sitting in the seats beside me. There was no mention of the debts of other people that Don assumed himself to help them get out from under their load. There was no mention of the forgiven rents and the properties Don financed himself for people he wanted to help through life. There was no mention of his faith and his belief in God, who gave his life purpose. There was no mention that he felt the greatest legacy he could give our children and grandchildren was for them to see his love for his wife and family in everyday life. His children did not know him, and I felt sorry that all they could honor him with were a few childish stories about themselves.

There was not one mention of Don's wife, except during the formal reading of the obituary from the newspaper, when the list of survivors was read. I was invisible. I did not exist. All of the eighteen years of love, life, and sharing our lives with others went to the grave with Don. The service ended with prerecorded country music, which was so out of character for Don that I was mortified. I was embarrassed that this was the last tribute to a man who was sophisticated and dignified. My husband deserved better.

The minister who gave the eulogy approached me after the funeral and lovingly offered his sympathy. He took my hands and said he wanted me to know I had been in his thoughts and prayers all week, and he was sorry he had not been able to contact me. He was so convincing that I felt sorry for him in the role to which he'd been assigned. The mystery of what he had been told and why he felt he could not even mention Don's wife weighed on my heart.

My friends and Don's friends were loving and compassionate and equally as embarrassed for me. Being shunned by Don's children did not go unnoticed by anyone. I could not understand how the family could stand the presence of one another after that so-called "tribute." There was an obvious line drawn at the mortuary that morning, as Don's children were completely separated from Don's friends and me. Alone, my son Rob made his way across the line to speak to Doug. He wanted to make sure Don's children knew how much my family loved Don and how much his life meant to my entire family and that we all shared in this deep grief.

The shrouded coffin was taken without a word out the back door of the mortuary. My husband's body was put in a hearse and taken forever away from me to be put in the ground in the dark red dirt of Oklahoma. I was not invited. The graveside service would be their reward and the fulfillment of all their actions; separation from his wife forever.

That afternoon, I watched the skies far to the southwest as a heavy dark thunderstorm settled over the country cemetery where my husband was being buried and then slowly rumbled toward me like a death march.

I was relieved to close the door at the mortuary and to that part of my life, and join my loving family and friends at my home. Alone late in the afternoon, I hid my face from the memories of the morning. I felt the fist that gripped my heart was tightening its hold on me. I prayed to have the strength to loose the grip of hatred and anger and to be free again to breathe. I hoped the "reign of terror" was over, and I would have no more dealings, ever, with these people.

In our bedroom is the cabinet where I displayed my collection of "widows"—the lonely pieces from broken sets—all these years. As I walked past it and my eyes fell on the many pieces that had outlasted their mates, I realized I had become of one of them. I was a widow.

There is a process one has to go through in grief. It was Don's time to go, so I did not mourn an interrupted life. I was thankful that he was free. He was gone for so long from me that I did not miss him. I did that grieving in the weeks after February 11, 2007. I realized only then that though I visited him every day, it was not the man I knew that I visited. I could not talk to him; reason with him; share my days and thoughts with him … or him with me.

I felt extreme sorrow. I was so sorry that this illness happened. I was sorry that Don was lost. I was sorry that he suffered. I was sorry for the lost time we planned to have together as we grew old. I was sorry for the mistakes we all made during this time. I was sorry that when he could have had the most comfort from my love, he doubted me.

An old friend called on me. She and her husband celebrated their fifty-fourth anniversary. She said being there to help each other grow old was the greatest blessing of their marriage. I said to her through tears, "That is what hurts me the most. That he was taken from me when he needed me the most." For that I was profoundly sorrowful. For weeks, my emotions were like an open sore; I wept if my eyes met others, and I wept when I was alone. I ached when I thought of Don; it was literally painful when I thought of his last year. I don't think there is much more we could have done to make a bigger, sadder mess of Don's last months with us.

I always felt I knew where we went when we died. Since Don's death, I cannot see clearly anymore. He's just gone; dead; nonexistent. What can his soul know? Where can he be? How can he not love me anymore? If he exists anywhere, how could he not love me anymore?

Now he visits me in my dreams. Once I wrote a poem to Don that began, "I wake of a morning; you are faintly there with me for I have dreamed of you." Every time I awaken, he is faintly there with me. I am dreaming with the passion that nearly consumed us both. I am dreaming of looking into his soul and he into mine. I am dreaming with great emotion, and I wake feeling close to him.

I wake of a morning
You are faintly there with me
For I have dreamed of you.
I sigh in the cool of the morning air
And your presence grows stronger
Around me.
The day tolls on, and whatever I do,
Wherever I look
You are there in some form.
Sometimes I fight you away
'ere I should break and not be able to go on
for want of you.
When I lay my head upon my pillow
Loneliness for you engulfs me.
I wonder over minutes of your day;
Wonder if your thoughts have passed over me
If your voice called to me.
And I fall asleep, only to ...
Wake of a morning
And you are faintly there with me
For I have dreamed of you ....

My Personal Living Will

To my beloved son, Rob
 The purpose of this epistle is to state how I would and wouldn't like to die ... I could sum it up very briefly: The quicker, the better.

I don't want you to take this event of dying too seriously. I promise you, it's going to happen. So, why not make it a happy occasion?

You gave me joy and pride and, thank you very much, you rarely bored me.

Do not think that you should sustain any form of long-term care. It would weary you beyond endurance ... I do not want to financially impoverish you in any way. Money does not alter the inevitable.

It would not be life to me to not be able to feel your touch or know your smile. I don't want to exist confined to a room or small area, not watching the change of seasons, not breathing the good air or smelling the scent of the outdoors.

It would not be life if I could not recognize or remember you all and our lives together. I do not want to live past my time, which in some ways may be measured by the inability to contribute to my own physical needs because my mind is not able to function. We've both seen ghosts—bodies whose minds and souls are already gone. Do not cling to my body.

Do not resuscitate, do not put in a feeding tube, do not put me on a ventilator, do not torture me with any kind of so-called therapy, etc. Let me go. Just let me go. Even if you have to push a little. Call in hospice as soon as possible.

I prefer to be cremated. If I am cremated, it matters not where my ashes go. My soul belongs to God, and it is there that I will await you all to love throughout eternity. Do not fail me! Make sure your soul belongs to God also. Otherwise I have lived in vain, and eternity will be an awfully long time to want you.

As for a service: have a memorial party where no one cries, and everyone laughs. And do not play country music!

I have every confidence that all your decisions will be the right ones.

10 Things You Should Know about LBD

by LBDA 2008

Understanding Lewy Body Dementias

Lewy body dementias (LBD) affect an estimated 1.3 million individuals and their families in the United States. At the Lewy Body Dementia Association (LBDA), we understand that though many families are affected by this disease, few individuals and medical professionals are aware of the symptoms, diagnostic criteria, or even that LBD exists. There are important facts about Lewy body dementias that you should know if you, a loved one, or a patient you are treating may have LBD.

1. **Lewy body dementias (LBD) are the second most common form of degenerative dementia and is widely under-diagnosed:** The only other form of degenerative dementia that is more common than LBD is Alzheimer's disease (AD). Many individuals who have LBD are misdiagnosed, most commonly with Alzheimer's disease if they present with a memory disorder or Parkinson's disease if they present with movement problems.

2. **LBD can have three common presentations:** Some individuals will start out with a movement disorder leading to the diagnosis of Parkinson's disease and later develop dementia. Another group of individuals will start out with a memory disorder that may look like AD, but over time two or more distinctive features become apparent leading to the diagnosis of 'dementia with Lewy bodies' (DLB). Lastly, a small group will first present with neuropsychiatric symptoms, which can include hallucinations, behavioral problems, and difficulty with complex mental activities, leading to an initial diagnosis of DLB. Regardless of the initial symptom, over time all three presentations of LBD will develop very similar cognitive, physical, sleep and behavioral features, all caused by the presence of Lewy bodies throughout the brain.

3. **The most common symptoms of LBD include:**

    Dementia: problems with memory and thinking

    Hallucinations: seeing or hearing things that are not really present Cognitive fluctuations: unpredictable changes in concentration and attention

    Parkinson-like symptoms: rigidity or stiffness, shuffling gait, tremor, slowness of movement (bradykinesia)

    Severe sensitivity to neuroleptics (medications used to treat hallucinations)

    REM Sleep Behavior Disorder: a sleep disorder where people seemingly act out their dreams

4. **The symptoms of LBD are treatable:** Currently there are no medications approved specifically for the treatment of LBD. All medications prescribed for LBD are approved for a course of treatment for symptoms related to other diseases such as Alzheimer's disease and Parkinson's disease with dementia and offer symptomatic benefits for cognitive, movement and behavioral problems.

5. **Early and accurate diagnosis of LBD is essential:** Early and accurate diagnosis is important because LBD patients may react to certain medications differently than AD or PD patients. A variety of drugs, including anticholinergics and some antiparkinsonian medications, can worsen LBD symptoms. LBDA has compiled a list of medications that should be avoided.

6. **Traditional antipsychotic medications may be contraindicated for individuals living with LBD:** Many traditional antipsychotic medications (for example, Haldol, Mellaril) are commonly prescribed for individuals with Alzheimer's disease and other forms of dementia to control behavioral symptoms. However, LBD affects an individual's brain differently than other dementias. As a result, these medications can cause a severe worsening of movement and a potentially fatal condition known as neuroleptic malignant syndrome (NMS). NMS causes severe fever, muscle rigidity and breakdown that can lead to kidney failure.

7. **Early recognition, diagnosis and treatment of LBD can improve the patients' quality of life:** LBD may affect an individual's cognitive abilities, motor functions, and/or ability to complete activities of daily living. Treatment should always be monitored by your physician(s) and may include: prescriptive and other therapies, exercise, diet, sleep habits, changes in behavior and daily routines.

8. **Individuals and families living with LBD should not have to face this disease alone:** LBD affects every aspect of a person – their mood, the way they think, and the way they move. LBD patients and families will need considerable resources and assistance from healthcare professionals and agencies. The combination of cognitive, motor and behavioral symptoms creates a highly challenging set of demands for continuing care. LBDA was formed to help families address many of these challenges.

9. **Physician education is urgently needed:** An increasing number of general practitioners, neurologists, and other medical professionals are beginning to learn to recognize and differentiate the symptoms of LBD from other diseases. However, more education on the diagnosis and treatment of LBD is essential.

10. **More research is urgently needed!** Research needs include tools for early diagnosis, such as screening questionnaires, biomarkers, neuroimaging techniques, and more effective therapies. With further research, LBD may ultimately be treated and prevented through early detection and neuroprotective interventions. Currently, there is no specific test to diagnose LBD.

Lewy Body Dementia Association, Used with Permission